NLP

Dark Psychology in Neuro-linguistic
Programming, Mind Control, Persuasion, and
Reading People - Gain an Advantage over
Anyone

DEBORAH WEISS

Contents

Introduction

Congratulations on purchasing *NLP* and thank you for doing so.

The following chapters will discuss everything that you need to know when it comes to NLP and using it to get what you want. There are a lot of great things about NLP, but many people have a lot of misconceptions that come with NLP. There are some people even within the field of psychology who are against NLP and think that it is a bad thing. They worry that this tool, when put into the wrong hands, could end up causing more damage than good, even if it does end up benefiting the one who learns how to use it.

However, there is a lot of good that can come with the effective usage of NLP. NLP is something that helps you to learn more about the people around you. It helps you to learn how to read the body language of those near you, and to get what you want. Any tool, when put in the wrong hands, can be dangerous. But NLP is an effective tool that can do a lot of good, especially for the one who knows how to use it.

This guidebook is going to take some time to explore NLP and all of the parts that come with it. Inside, we are going to explore what NLP is, some of the controversies that come with NLP, and how you need to learn a bit of self-mastery before you stand a chance of learning how to use some of the tools of NLP on other people.

From there, we are going to move on to how NLP can influence the past, present, and future of you and of your intended target, how to start using NLP against someone else, and even a bit of information on some of the techniques that you can use, and how you can take what you want from others without having to apologize all of the time. We will also spend some time talking about the morality of using NLP, and why these morals, and the values of society, maybe shouldn't be an important consideration when it comes to figuring out whether or not you should use NLP for your own needs.

There are so many great benefits that can come from using NLP in your own life. It allows you to learn how to work with other people, how to read what other people are thinking and meaning, and ensures that you are able to get more of what you want and need out of life. When you are ready to learn more about NLP, especially dark NLP, and how to use it in your own life, make sure to check out this guidebook to help you get started.

There are plenty of books on this subject on the market, thanks again for choosing this one! Every effort was made to ensure it is full of as much useful information as possible, please enjoy!

What are the Foundations of NLP?

The get an understanding of dark NLP on a theoretical level, you first need to have a good understanding of the ideas that come with NLP, and what it is based on. NLP began when two people developed a set of ideas that looked into human behavior and how it could be influenced. Their ideas soon became known as neurolinguistic programming, more commonly known as NLP. While the techniques that went with NLP were first unknown, they started to get more exposure through the years. Many people know about NLP and what it is all about, but very people really know how to apply the techniques.

NLP comes with three main areas, looking at the way that ideas are filtered. These three areas include learning, subjectivity, and consciousness. NLP is going to teach that there isn't an absolute or objective understanding of the world around us, and instead, each person is going to work to form their own picture of the world. This picture is going to vary from one person to another and each one is going to consist of data that comes in through the five senses, and the language that the person attaches to this data.

It is theorized that this combination of descriptive language and sensory input is going to be what leads to behaviors that are either effective according to the subjective map of the world, or they become maladaptive and harmful to our own pursuits and our own aims.

One area where those who look into NLP are pretty much in the agreement is where it has a good understanding of the human mind as having both a conscious and an unconscious dimension. And most of the teaching that you see with NLP is that it is on the belief that a lot of influence is going to occur on the subconscious level. What this means is that we can often be manipulated and influenced on a level that they won't really be able to see.

NLP is going to see people as behaving in ways that go with the three key aspects, mainly the why, the how, and the what. The what is going to focus on the external behavior and the physiology a person exhibits in a given situation. Then the how is going to deal with some of the thinking patterns that the person has internally and are going to govern their own patterns of decision making. And then the why is going to deal with the supporting beliefs, values, and assumptions that point a person in one direction instead of another one.

If you are supposed to fully understand the three aspects that are part of NLP, then you will be able to effectively model the complete reality of someone else's behavior. It is important to note that it is the internal process that is being copied, and this is going to be what will lead to the external behavior, rather than just crudely mimicking the external behavior on its own. Without both the internal and external parts, the behavior that you are trying to work with is going to look pretty phony and insincere.

Advocates of NLP are going to beyond just passively accepting these factors, the ones that are going to compromise the behavior of the person. Instead, it advocates that there needs to be an active exploration of it and how it is going to be able to manipulate the variables at hand. When this happens, there is a better understanding of the relationship between each and which ones are going to be the most essential to achieve the desired results.

Now, you will find that there is a big contrast between the NLP model of understanding behavior and the traditional way of looking at behavior. Traditionally, we are going to start taking on a new behavior by learning one piece of a skill at a time, and then all of these little parts are going to add up and form a new behavior. When we are looking at NLP, you will find that it goes the other way. the person is going to be presented with all of the components of the behavior at once, and then they will start to subtract out the different parts until they are able to have just the essential aspects.

This is a process that is going to simplify behaviors and then reducing them to only their crucial aspects is similar to the business process which aims to map out a series of steps and identify which are essential and which are not. When we are looking at this sense, the process of refining behaviors with the help of applying NLP, and this is a way for you to ensure personal efficiency.

NLP also concerns itself with the question of finding the difference between the two types of people within any given field, those who succeed and those who don't. Success modeling seeks to find exactly what other people who were successful and compared it to the things that unsuccessful people have done. Then you can choose to avoid the right things, and follow the right tasks, to get the results that you want.

The main outlook of this NLP is going to be summarized as simplifying and identifying the actors that can lead to success in a situation as a simple process model. When this model has been identified and simplified it can be applied in order to get drastic amounts of results in a short amount of time, especially when it is compared to the traditional way of doing things.

One of the key ideas that are behind working with what is

known as dark NLP is that human beings are going to lack any kind of concrete identity, which is going to make them more at risk for the influence that others try to put on them, whether that is a good thing or a bad thing will depend on who tries to mold that person.

Traditional NLP is going to take this idea of the identity as being fluid, and then I am used as a basis so that therapists are able to help people overcome some of the major roadblocks that may be holding them back in a lie. But with the dark LP, this fluidity of identity is going to mean that a person can be manipulated based on the will of others. Because there is the potential or some influence that is more malicious, it is important to understand more about how NLP works and how to avoid becoming the victim in these scenarios.

Dark psychology is also going to understand that most of the time, humans are going to be less in control of their own free will than they like to believe. For example, the majority of people, when they were asked, will report that they often feel like they are entirely in control of their own thought processes, and they state that they would not obey a command or instructions that happen to go against this kind of free will. But the studies show that this is not necessarily true.

One of the classic experiments that have been done in psychology, and has had a direct influence on the concepts of dark psychology, can shatter this illusion and helps to show that we are often not as in control as we like to think we are. In the famous Milgram study, there were volunteers who would need to administer electric shocks when the wrong answer was given or a learning test. During this, the majority of those who were told to do these shocks would continue to do it, even if they could hear the screams of those who were being punished.

With the experiment above, we can see that people seem to have the obedience to authority that is inherent, and they are less free and have less free will than they tend to assume.

In another study, known as the Zimbardo experiment, there is an insight into another aspect that has gone along with dark psychology for some time, which is the willingness of humans to assume behaviors based on what their role is for that situation. In this experiment, the participants were going to be divided up in a random order to either be prisoners or prison guards. Those who were in the role of a prison guard were more and more willing to carry on acts of cruelty and even to abuse their power the longer that the experiment went on.

When these two studies are taken together, they are going to offer two big concepts, which are also going to be the core principles that come with dark psychology. These concepts show that people can easily be led by others and that behaviors can be influenced in more than one way. This is something that can be seen as disturbing for most people, and they may choose to ignore it. Those who believe it are in the minority, and they are often willing to exploit these ideas, which place them in a unique situation to take advantage of others to their own ends.

Another thing that we need to take a look at with dark psychology is the idea of priming. Priming states that there are a lot of factors that can influence people, and many of these factors are going to be outside the perception of that person. For example, the choice of language that one person is using towards their target has been shown to influence the speed at which they will move after the fact. In addition, words that sound similar to other words can sometimes be used by the manipulator in order to plant ideas into that person's mind, without them having an idea that these thoughts have been planted.

Dark psychology is also going to exploit the tendency of most humans to be really susceptible to the opinion of the majority, even if this kind of influence happens to go against the own perception and rationality of the target. This was shown in a series of experiments who found that subjects would easily change their own ideas about something when they had some influence by the group majority.

This is a concept that is going to be used by some cults and groups with extremist ideologies. They may use this as a way to brainwash those they want to influence. When someone is surrounded by people who have certain opinions and views, they will not only start to believe what they have heard but often they will gain the feeling that they did change of their own free will, rather than changing because of force or influence.

A willingness to accept

As anyone in psychological research will tell you, a key part of making sure that the research is successful is the ability to accept what the evidence is showing you, rather than trying to go through and seek out ways to confirm the theories that you already have. This concept is going to apply to the individual pursuit of dark NLP as well, because you will need to be willing to accept that what works, actually does work. Of course, the results may not be exactly what you had hoped, and you may not like what it is telling you about people, but it is the truth.

The willingness to accept can also extend out to the times where you will need to take a look at yourself and some of the choices you made in the past. There is no point, and it certainly isn't going to help you, to shy away from seeing things in a brutally honest manner. You will find that this guidebook is going to emphasize the importance of moving away from the idea of judging yourself, and instead find a way to accept yourself.

We have all gone through and done things that we are not proud of. We maybe went along with a mob mentality at some point and did things that were obviously against our values. We may have inflicted more harm to others than was needed because we were told to do so by an authority figure.

This is a part of life and is a good example of how NLP can be used against you and other people.

Letting go of the preconceived notions that you have about mankind and how they behave, and even letting go of the judgments that you have against yourself, will make a bit of difference in how well you can learn about, and use, the ideas of NLP.

The red pill

As we go through on this guidebook and learn more about dark NLP, it is important to understand that no one has an identity that is fixed. Each person is able to be influenced, and with all of the different influences in our lives, it is common to see them change on a regular basis. For some people, changing their beliefs is going to be easier to adopt than it is for some of the others. It can be upsetting because it often means that we don't have all the control in life that we wish we did. But it can also be a bit liberating because it means that each of us has the freedom necessary to reinvent ourselves at any stage of life that we choose. We are never too young or too old, we can go through and make the changes that we want in our lives.

Here it is also important that we learn how to embrace the fact that what we consider as conventional morality is just an illusion, and people are actually willing to perform a variety of acts that will go against what is seen as moral in their culture if there is some benefit to them for doing this. It doesn't matter what the morals are and how closely the person may have said they were going to follow the morals in the past. The fact remains that if they think it is going to benefit them to act in a different manner, they will.

The next thing that we need to understand is that morality is actually something that is relative, and there isn't a standard that exists. Although we are able to see some prohibitions that are common through any different cultures, there isn't going to be a universal standard of morality out there. indeed, these similarities can be explained that they are in accordance with the theory of evolution from Darwin. This states that if something is found to be useful when it comes to the survival of the species, then it is going to be incorporated into the moral norms for that time.

In many cases, dark NLP is going to encourage you, or even open up the mind, to the idea of operating in a way that is different than what you have been taught at church or through other forms of social influence. One example that is commonly occurring is the teaching of NLP going against many of the Christian teachings. When you do a closer examination here, it shows that while the Christians teach that it is praiseworthy to be meek, this is meant to be a form of social control. On the other hand, the dark NLP is going to teach us how to empower others to shamelessly pursue what they want out of life. The first is going to make people passive and easier to control, and the latter is going to benefit the individual directly.

There is also no way to escape the idea that dark NLP is going to ask you to go against the common view that people do work well together and all interactions need to be viewed as collaborative opportunities with others. With dark NLP, you are going to learn that each interaction needs to be viewed as a sort of zero-sum, where one party is going to win and the other will lose.

There is a lot of things that dark NLP is going to go against. Mainly, you must have a willingness to see that acting your own self-interest is not something that has to be immoral. In fact, over time you will find that the idea of morals is fluid and ever-changing, and this means that it is not a good thing to base your decisions on. This is why many of those who practice dark NLP will choose to base their decisions just on self-interest, rather than worrying so much about morality. This is the best way to consistently guarantee that the outcome you get for your choices is going to work in your own favor.

Predator or prey

Net, the variety of applied examples will help to show how you can put into practice the ideas of dark NLP and can ensure that you have a clear advantage in the different situations that you may find yourself when using NLP. This is going to be highlighted through the use of predator or prey. What this means is that in any social interaction that you partake in, there is going to be one person who is acting, and the other person, or the prey, is the one who is being acted upon.

Imagine that you are going through an appraisal or some kind of assessment in your professional life. In this kind of situation, there are two ways that you are able to handle it; you can either be the one who takes the decisive action, or you can risk that someone else is going to act on you. This can make a big difference in how your appraisal goes and what settings for targets that you will need to meet in the upcoming year.

To start, let's say that the assessment starts out with a discussion on how well you performed over the past year. You can either sit there and passively accept how the assessor talks about your performance. Or you can take the reins and highlight some of your own achievements, ensuring that your performance is shown in as good of a light as possible. If you let the assessor go over things, they may or may not read things out in your favor. And they are certainly going to at least spend a little time bringing up the things that went wrong, or the things that you underperformed with.

If you take the reins here, you can learn how to gloss over certain things, and minimize the negative. Each of us has some things that maybe didn't go the right way throughout the year, but this doesn't mean that we did poorly at our jobs. But that is just how the assessor may see things. They may focus on the negative as a way to make you take on more work or to refuse to give you a bonus. But that is only if you let them be the ones in charge. If you use NLP and take control, and work to explain all of the good, and twist the negative into something good, you will be the one in control and able to get what you want.

It is important for you to keep the idea of predator and prey in mind during any interactions that you have in terms of romance in your life as well. There are many times when one partner in the relationship simply wants to exploit the other one. By filtering this truth through the lends of a filter for predator or prey, we will see that these people are trying to make us a prey, and they don't really have the best intentions in place, even if they get in a relationship with us that seems romantic.

Always be wary of the idea that you could be pretty for someone else. This helps you to be guarded at all times and can protect you from naively slipping into a trap that someone else has set. You are the one who wants to be in charge, the predator, not someone else. Always being on the lookout for this, rather than just assuming that everyone is nice and has your best interests at heart, can help you to get more of what you want out of life.

2

Why Has NLP Gotten Such a Bad Reputation?

Why Has NLP Gotten Such a Bad Reputation?

Now that we have taken a little look at NLP and some of the basics that come with it, it is time to work in more detail and understand more about what it is, how to make it work, and so much more. When we look in the real world, we are going to see that NLP is a highly challenged way of thinking. It goes against the main morality standards, and the social norms, of our culture, and this means that there may be a bit of backlash with using it.

This chapter is going to spend some time going through several real-life examples of NLP and how it has the power to make some changes to your life, sometimes for the better and sometimes for the worse. We will even take a look at some of the uses of NLP that are the darkest and the most controversial, and because of this, there is a lot of issues and naysayers when it comes to NLP. Understanding these controversies and more will make you more effective when it comes to using NLP in your own lie.

How powerful is NLP, some real-life examples

At this point, we will need to look at a range of insights into the power that NLP has to influence lives. We are not going to waste our time with the moral stance on NLP because we are going to spend more time learning how to use these techniques in order to gain more power through NLP, as long as it is used in an effective manner. Let's get started.

One powerful example that comes with NLP is how it can be used in order to cure people of a negative condition. One story of this is a man who decided to visit a therapist of NLP, with the complaint that he wasn't able to give up smoking cigarettes. Even though this habit had resulted in some negative health effects, and this habit cost him a lot of money (he was up to three packs each day), the man had been unable to find the right tools or the right motivation to get the habit to go away.

The therapist was able to help. Using the ideas of NLP, the therapist was able to use a series of envisioning techniques in order to make some changes to the view that the man had when thinking about smoking. Instead of seeing the cigarettes as a type of guilty pleasure that he was allowed to enjoy, the man was able to swap out the imagery of cigarettes with that of bad health and death, because the therapist was able to manipulate the internal viewpoint of the man, that man was able to quit because he no longer had a desire for the cigarettes.

That is just one example though. The next story that we are going to take a look at concerning NLP is going to come from the world of business. In this story, one high-ranking executive who was in the European division of a technology company was summoned to go to a meeting with another executive, one who is often intimidating to others and who was in America. Although this woman executive was respected inside her own division of the company, she had achieved this by being supportive and likable to the others in the division as well. She didn't really have a lot of assertion in her, and this made her fearful of meeting with the American executive.

Due of these issues, the woman decides that she needs to visit with an NLP teacher to help her learn a few ways to become more comfortable and more confident when it was time to meet in America. She was taught one of the techniques of NLP that is known as anchoring, which is where you learned how to link back emotion to some kind of physical trigger.

For this example, the woman was taught to think back through the history of her life, to a tie where you had gained total confidence and in control over the situation that was taking place. The woman was able to do this. Next, she was instructed to link this feeling with colored light. Once she picked out the colored light in her mind, she would then move the colored light over to the floor in front of her, and use it to draw a big circle that went all the way around her. This was able to provide that woman with a very big feeling of confidence and security, as long as she remembered the boundaries of the circle.

When the woman had to head to her meeting in America, she was able to work with this technique and found a way to get rid of the fears that she had been dealing with while interacting with that executive. During the meeting, she was able to calmly and collectedly deal with any situation that came out. In the end, it turned out that this executive just wanted to discuss a strategy with her, and she was never disciplined or criticized during that meeting. But because she took the time to work with NLP training, this woman executive was able to avoid experiencing all the worry and stress that she would have otherwise.

One of the most controversial ways that the process of NLP has been used is when they are trying to start a new romantic relationship. There are a few different schools of thought that have been dedicated solely on their ability to teach a form of seduction that is based on NLP, and we will take a look at this topic in more depth later on. For now, we will just focus on a brief insight to help us get started.

One of the most well-known teachers of NLP currently

runs seminars to help mean learn how to use NLP to induce good feelings in members of the opposite sex. The idea is that when the men are able to do this, they are going to increase their chances of having a successful romantic encounter with that woman. The methods are going to revolve around the ideas of generating a positive internal state that can then be passed on to the other person with the idea of the law of the state of transference.

The idea behind this and the ways that you are able to carry it out on your chosen target are going to be outlined a bit later. But you will find that if you are able to induce some good feelings with the other person, so they are more likely to enter into the relationship with you.

Of course, with the examples that we have just looked at, we are taking a look at some of the more positive, and sometimes more accepted, uses of NLP in the life of the person. There are some more options that you can work with, some that may seem a bit sinister and others that are harmful and even hurtful to the target you have chosen.

Darker examples of NLP in the real world

One darker area where NLP can be applied is with influence. While the majority of people who use NLP are going to use it to help enhance their success in the dating world, there are those who have devoted themselves to learning some darker applications when it comes to what you can do with the process of NLP. These are generally not accepted as part of the social norms and morals, but they can ensure that the predator is able to get what they want.

Patterns can be one of the techniques of dark NLP that can be used to seduce. A series of patterns gained notoriety when you are in the community of seduction, and they are now known as the banned patterns. The reason that these patterns earned their name is because they are seen as too amoral and too dark for most in the community to accept.

Since these patterns are going to have a good deal of notoriety with them, they are going to be sought out in some way or another by the community. But they are still going to be hard to find. These patterns are going to be presented in this section so that you can see how the good NLP and the dark NLP are similar, and how they are going to be different.

One of the patterns that fall into dark NLP is going to be called the shadow and the rising sun. This is one that is often put with the seduction community because it is going to draw upon some of the ideas that are found in the Jungian psychology, where it is going to work to unlock some of the dark sides of women, the hidden parts that come with her personality. This one is going to be achieved by the seducer talking about the idea of contrasts. They are focusing on talking just about imagery that contrasts, in order to show off the idea of darkness as light and dark, day and night, and yin and yang.

The seducer is going to take this even further by talking

about how each person has their own dark side and how this is the idea of a rising sun that still casts a shadow with it. The seducer can then invite their target to step into their own dark side and to start accepting and viewing the world with this new lens. This is going to help put the target into a state of more susceptibility, where they may be willing to act in a way that they wouldn't do in other circumstances.

Another kind of technique that can be used is going to be done along with the above technique, but some things are going to be changed around. This one is known as the hospital pattern. With this pattern, the seducer is going to work to fluctuate the emotional state of the target between extremes, either extreme pleasure or extreme pain, and it is going to rapidly change between the two at regular intervals.

This rapid change of emotional states, which will go between the extremes multiple times, is going to help to make it so that the target feels unstable with their emotions, which makes them more susceptible to the influence. When the target reaches this new susceptible state, the seducer would then be able to anchor the perception of the target in any manner that they wish. They will usually make sure that the feelings of the target are going to be turned to feel immense pleasure with the seducer, which allows the seducer to trigger these kinds of feelings on demand.

Another dark usage of NLP is going to be with a pattern interrupt. This is when the seducer will use some of their dark NP in order to stop the actions of the target, and they want to reduce the defense mechanisms and rationality of their target as much as possible.

For example, if the target is talking to their seducer and they begin to list off some of the logical reasons why it doesn't make sense to be with the seducer any longer, when the seducer is going to try and distract them a bit and get their mind on something else entirely. They may say something like "what is your favorite color?" This stops the thought process of the target and can stop their defense mechanisms at the same time.

NLP has on occasion been used in more of a dark way to make it so that the target begins to question which memories they have that are real, and which ones may have been fabricated along the way. there are techniques out there that are going to put the target into a state of relaxation so they float between being awake and being asleep. This works for the seducer because the target is going to be highly suggestible during that time.

Both of the above can be used by the seducer in order to disrupt the feelings of identity that the target has. This causes the target to question the different values and beliefs that they have about who they are. This is sometimes what is used as the first step in brainwashing when you want to make sure that the target is a blank slate and that you are able to fill it in with what you want.

You can work with a similar technique in order to implant

some false memories into the mind of your target and make them feel real. Just like with the last technique, the target is going to be placed into a state of deep relaxation, which makes them more susceptible to influence. They will be led back through the memories, and at the right point, the target will be asked some leading questions into remembering something that most likely didn't happen. It will start out with a real memory, but then the seducer will try to make some changes to turn that memory into something else.

The controversy that comes with NLP

After hearing about some of the different forms of NLP that have been used in the past, it is no hard to imagine why it has garnered such a bad reputation over the years. NLP is actually one of the most controversial parts of psychology today. There are a lot of different controversies that have come with NLP, which is why there are so many people who are concerned that this form of mind control and way of doing things may not be the best because it isn't in the best interest of the target.

To start, some of the earliest forms and criticisms of NLP came from the mainstream psychology profession. Traditional therapists and psychologists stated that the process of NLP was dangerous because it was taking shortcuts in order to get the results, results that should take a much longer time to accomplish. According to many in the field, taking these kinds of shortcuts mean that the individuals weren't really healed and many believed that the patients simply learned how to hide their traumas deeper than ever before.

Another controversy that often showed up is the idea that NLP seemed to encourage people to act in an immoral way. because NLP is going to teach participants how to act in a way that can influence others, it is sometimes seen as a way to encourage others to act in ways that are selfish and detrimental. NLP teachers hi back saying that this is unfair and that almost any thought from the school of psychology could be used for good and for bad, so NLP should not be singled out.

For those in more feminist circles, there is criticism that NLP is used as a form of seduction. These groups believe that NLP is going to take away the element of choice and they are going to make one or the other of these partners do something that they wouldn't agree to do in a normal circumstance. The counter-argument to this is that, when it is used properly, NLP can actually enhance the romantic encounter and that it is able to help people experience a greater range of positive emotions when they are with the other person.

The way that NLP has been taught over the years has been criticized as well. It is alleged that the environment for NLP is going to be taught is similar to what is found in a cult setting. Those who are being taught these thoughts are supposed to accept the principles of NLP without any kind of questions.

There are some counter-arguments to this as well as schools who teach **NLP** insist that those who are learning about **NLP** are allowed and encouraged to believe or not believe the things that they are taught, and that the teachers of **NLP** have no means to suppress the free thoughts of the students. And they insist that those who receive the certification for **NLP** are only going to get it when they are truly ready.

3

Become the Master Before Attempting to Master Others

N ow, before we start to dive more into the idea of NLP and how it is used, we first need to explore the idea of self-mastery. If you don't have a good mastery of yourself before jumping into all of this, then there is no hope that you will be able to master the thoughts, feelings, and emotions of another person. We are going to take a look at the importance of self-mastery, what this means, and how you can learn to control yourself so that it is much easier to start controlling other people with NLP.

Know your outcomes

The first key that we need to take a look at when it comes to mastering ourselves is to know what you want, no matter what the situation is about. If you have no idea what you are aiming for, it is impossible to know which strategy is going to be the best, and which one you should pursue. Always go into a situation with a good and clear objective in mind. Realize that any kind of objective, even if it is not perfect, is going to be better than having no objective in place at all. You do have the option to adjust your goals and refine them as you go, but at least start out with some kind of goal in mind.

It is important that you make the intended outcome, also known as your target, as specific and clear as possible. You will be able to do this as you go along and learn what works for you. But you never want to make the goals too vague, even in the beginning, because then it is impossible to measure these goals, and how can you assess how far you have come. Make sure that when you are picking your goals, you go with something that is definitive, which you can measure the progress for, and which has an ending that is clear.

Know your drives

Knowing what outcome you want to get out of the situation is a good first step when you are trying to work on self-mastery. But it isn't the last step. Without taking the time to know your deepest drives and the things that motivate you to take some massive actions right here and now, it is impossible for you to reach your outcome in an effective way.

To start with, you should sit down and write out anything that comes to your mind when you are thinking about the things that motivate you. Don't question yourself or make any judgments during this time; just spend some time writing down anything that comes to your mind. When you are done and can't come up with anything new to put here, then you can put down the pen and stop writing. Now there is a list of different ideas and topics in front of you. Go through and rank each one based on which one gives you the most motivated, what gives you the second motivation, and so down.

You can then list out the three top motivators, the ones that you feel the most motivation from and you want to concentrate your energy on now. You should write these out on their own piece of paper, going in order from the highest to the lowest. You can then link these three drives back to the outcome that we talked about before. You can then start to see how your goal is going to relate back to those drives. And overall, this is going to ensure that you have the right motivation tied back to the goals, and you are more likely to work hard to reach those goals.

Know your values

At this point, you have now gone through and established your intended outcome, and then linked it back to one of the main things that will motivate your lie. This is very powerful, but to make sure that you can really increase your self-mastery to a new level, you will need to establish your values and then link them back to the intended outcome as well.

There is no point in us taking the time to suggest which values you would like to consider because this is a very personal topic. Just think about the things in life that are going to matter the most to you. And then write down the values that are going to be unable to help you keep those things. Once you have been able to establish all of the major values, take some time to rank them from the most powerful to the lead powerful, just like we did with the drives earlier. Once you have your top three values figured out, you can write them down on their own pieces of paper.

Just like what we did with the drivers earlier, you will want to go through and link your values into not only your outcome but also to your drives. You want to ensure that all of these factors are going to be in alignment, to ensure that you are focused on a deep and a subconscious level to achieve your own outcome. This may take a bit more time to accomplish, but it really does some wonders when it comes to ensuring that all of your motivations are going to reinforce each other, and keeps you away from isolating each one.

Your motivation can be temporary, but your habits are not

To make sure that you are able to achieve your intended outcome, you must make sure that you fully understand your values and drives. To motivate yourself about the outcome that you want, you must think about all of the ways that you are going to feel once you have been able to achieve that goal. For example, if your goal is to get that big promotion at work, imagine how you are going to feel, and what will change in your life, once you actually get for that promotion.

Once you have a clear idea of what your goal is and what achieving that goal is going to mean for you, you will find that it is much easier to stay motivated and to control yourself in order to reach that goal. However, motivation is easier to attain that it is to keep around for a long time. That's way, once you have your motivation, you should use it to help you build up the proper habits that are needed to support the outcome. If you don't make that effort now, you will end u falling into patterns that don't support your values and your influence in life.

Let's look at an example of this. To form a budget, you will need to form the habits of recording your spending for a period of time, adding up all that you have to spend, and then split it up between the different categories. You need to get into the habit of looking for ways to cut back on spendings, such as always going with special offers or generic options at the store. You can even form the habit of balancing your budget against your income to make sure you are reaching your goals.

It isn't enough for you to just establish some habits, and have motivations in place, but they are done in isolation. It is so important that you are able to link them together. You can do this by ensuring you link the motivation to the habits that you want to carry out on a regular basis. You may find that the anchoring technique from NLP can work for this. For this one, you would trigger your state of motivation by envisioning the good feelings that are triggered when you achieve the goal. You would then use a repeated physical gesture, such as touching your wrist when you carry out the routine habit.

Using this gesture is going to link the feeling of motivation to your physical gesture. You can then trigger this motivation just by doing the physical trigger. It is that easy. Once you have had the time to create these habits, you are going to keep going through and following through with them, even when you have lost out on some of the motivation. There are going to be days that are tough and days when your motivation is going to be very low. But if you develop the habits early on, you will continue to work towards your goals, and you will achieve them, even when things aren't as easy as they once were.

One of the hardest things to work on when it is time to start working with NLP is to learn how to master yourself. Once you have mastered how to handle all of the goals and dreams of your own, then you will have more control over dealing with control over others.

4

Is It Possible to Take Control of Others?

N ow that we have taken the time to understand ourselves through the principles of NLP to understand and leverage your own outcomes, drives, and values, you will be shown how to extend this kind of self-mastery and use it to take control over others. You will learn the right techniques that are going to make it easier to understand what makes a person act in a certain way, and then you can learn how to influence them through your words and actions.

One thing to keep in mind is that you should make sure that there is some caution with the techniques that you are using. They are going to be really powerful techniques, and the power that you can gain with this can't be overstated. Let's take a look at some of the steps that you can do in order to take control of others with the help of NLP.

Hacking the secret blueprint of anyone

The first step that you need to use in order to gain a level of influence over someone is to figure out what their secret blueprint is that makes them who they are as a person. There are going to be several aspects of a person you need to understand in order to gain control over them that you want. This blueprint is going to show you their doubts, hopes, fears, and the things that they like and dislikes about themselves. You will now be shown how to figure out all of these aspects of a person's blueprint and how to take action based on this information to increase the amount of influence you have over the other person.

To help you understand more about the fears that someone has, there are two main methods that work the best for that. These can either be used on their own or in conjunction. The first method that we can take a look at is the passive method. This method is just going to involve you simply paying close attention to the other person, listening to how they talk, and what they talk about, in order to determine the things that worry them the most.

You will find that different people are more or less obvious in the way that they reveal this aspect of themselves. Some people talk about things and clearly state they are worried by them, while others are not really all that explicit about it, and instead they are going to use some hints at it with the general demeanor and tone of voice that they use when it is time to discuss certain issues.

The second method that you can use is a more active method. For this one, you can listen for a bit, and then try to lead the other person to the responses that you are looking for. For example, you could causally lead the conversation over to the topic of health with a particular person. Depending on how willing the other person is to talking about the topic, their tone of voice, and how physically comfortable they are with it, you will be able to figure out how much that particular person worries about health. You can use it for any topic in order to gauge the fear that the person has on that issue.

Uncovering the hopes of another person is often going to be easier than determining the fears that they have. This is because you will find that people are more willing to disclose their hopes rather than their fears. Many people like to give away what they aspire to in life by disclosing their aims for the future. Even some of the aspects that seem trivial amount a person, such as the purchases that they choose to make, can indicate the way that they are going to see themselves, and how they like to be seen by others.

If you are looking to encourage others to open up about their hopes is to start talking about some of the hopes that you have. This can help make it so that the other person feels more candid. A manipulative and dark NLP spin that you can use is to disclose some of your hopes, ones that aren't sincere, that are specifically intended to increase the comfort level towards a certain topic. For example, if you tell the other person that you have some money worries, even though you don't have those money worries. This makes the target feel that money worries is acceptable to talk about, and they will then open up to you.

There are a lot of things that you can use when it comes to how you can use this same idea to manipulate the other person. You can use the things that the person likes and dislikes about life, they could lower the self-esteem of the other person by insulting them in a subtle way, and can play the fears against them. You can look at their dreams, their hopes, the things they are afraid of and more. You are able to observe the other person to determine what makes them tick and how you can best manipulate them.

How to read what is in the other person's eyes

If it is true that the eyes are the windows to the soul, then this is definitely something that you need to consider when trying to use NLP on another person. To begin reading the eye movements of another person, it is important to ask a series of questions and make a mental note of the direction of the eye movement as they answer. Start by asking the person something that is factual, one that you know they are going to answer in a truthful manner. You could ask their name or the date of their birth. Pay attention to where they look. This lets you know which direction they are going when they are telling the truth. Then, if they go in a different direction, they will most likely be telling you a lie.

Finally, you should ask a question that you are hoping to get a lie out of the other person. So, if you know that this person is pretty insecure about the salary that they make, ask them if they make a figure that is a bit higher than what you are sure they make. There is a high chance that they are going to agree with you because they won't want to reveal the lower amount that they are insecure about. The movement that the eyes are going to make, as well as the tone that is in that person's voice, will help you to detect if there is something that they are lying about in the future.

Linguistic mind control

You will also find that the choice of language that the other person chooses to use is going to be a really powerful indicator of what drives them, as well as how they see the world. For example, there are those who are going to show that they agree with you by saying something like "that feels right" "I know what you mean" or "I hear you". Their choice of language is going to show how they perceive the world, and whether that is through their logic, touch, or sight. When you know what the perception is for that person, you can then draw upon that and explain ideas you wish them to disagree with in a language that isn't in alignment with that system.

You will also find that by listening to the other person, they are going to start disclosing words that have a special level of meaning or some significance for them. For example, you may find that when the person is talking about someone they have a lot of admiration for, they may use the word brilliant. And this word is only going to show up when their emotions are heightened. This is a good sign that the word has some kind of significance to that person. You can then use this information to your advantage and deploy the word in some of the statements that you make in order to trigger an agreement from the other person. Make sure that it is used sparingly though. If you overuse it, this is going to seem obvious and can come across as an unnatural thing.

Often the choice of words that the person chooses to go with is going to change when their internal state is different. The more that you are around the other person, the easier it will be to figure out what words are used for each different internal voice of that person. This is useful because you are then able to modify your own choice of words and behavior to ensure that it is compatible with that person's world view at that time.

The power of mirroring someone else

The first thing that you can do to make sure that you are able to take control of someone physically, as well as with their inner state is to really take note of their body language. You need to always take a constant amount of notice of the people you interact with, and the way that they will move, hold themselves, their expressions, where their feet are positions, and how they move their hands, the smaller the detail, the better.

Once you have a good idea of the body language that the person likes to use, you are then able to mimic them as well. You don't want to do this too much, but using it a little bit is going to make a big difference in how the other person is able to react to you. If you use the same tone of voice, if you can move your hands in a similar way, and if you can copy some of the little habits that they have, they are instantly going to feel a new connection with you.

There are a few ways that you can double check to see if you have built up the amount and type of rapport that you want with your target. Of course, the main method to look at is through physical leading, which we will talk about a bit more in a moment. Some of the things that are going to become apparent after you have been able to mirror the other person effectively is that the target is going to find it easier to open up and talk with you. They are going to have an emotional tone that is warmer, and they may disclose more information. They may even agree with your opinions more because they feel that connection with you.

Using leading and pacing to take control

One of the most effective ways that you can check whether your mirroring efforts have worked and if they created a sense of connection is to see if you can physically take control of the interaction with your target. But how are you supposed to be able to do this?

The first stage of the process is to spend a period of time

mirroring someone. You want to copy, in a subtle manner, any changes in the body language of that target so that they feel comfortable and like the two of you are on the same page. Then, after you do this for some time, you can make a little change in your own body language. You could make it as simple as moving where your right hand is. if you are successful, you will find that your target is going to start copying the body language that you did.

When someone starts to copy the changes that you are showing in your own body languages, this means that they have fallen deep into the rapport that you have set up, and they are ready to be led by you. This means that it is the prime time for you to get them to agree with what you are saying, or to get them to carry out any other kind of manipulation that you want.

If you find that you try out this step to lead the interaction, and the other person doesn't start to copy you, this doesn't mean that all is lost at this point. It may mean that you tried to move ahead too quickly, and you just need to mirror them a bit longer. It can sometimes take a bit longer with some people compared to others, and you need to just give it the time that is needed. Eventually, you are going to have enough of this rapport going on in the subconscious that they will start to follow your lead.

The key to being able to lead someone effectively in this manner is to start out by making some small leads before gradually working your way up to make some of the bigger changes that are needed with your body language. For example, you could start out with a rather small change of moving the position of just the hand. Then build up to moving the entire arm. And then move both arms, or do some other bold movement at this time.

The greater the mirroring level that the target shows, the greater the rapport that you have built up with them. And once you have reached this level, it means that you are now able to influence them on the corresponding event that you would like.

5

Don't Control the Present, Control the Past and Future As Well

One of the things that you will see as the most powerful aspects of NLP is the ability that it gives the user to control all of the personal dimensions that come with time including the past, the present, and the future. Many of the techniques for personal and self-help in the world today are going to make a halfhearted attempt to focus on just one of the above aspects at a time. For example, they may try to promote a better today, or a more hopeful tomorrow. But when you are working with the ideas and principles that come with dark NLP, you won't be limited so much on this kind of outlook. Because the principles are going to be grounded in reliable scientific evidence, it is as effective in one time as in any other.

In this chapter, we are first going to take a look at how you can see the world by looking at it in the lens of dark NLP.

Some of the classic NLP concepts will be updated and refined in light of the latest dark psychology discoveries, and we are going to spend some time taking a deeper look at them to see how they are able to change the way we view the world.

How to see the world with dark NLP

The first key to understanding that the user of dark NLP needs to reach is that it doesn't matter as much about what you say or do, what matters is the result that you are able to get out of this process. This means that the process is going to be very tactical and results oriented. The dark NLP way of viewing the world is going to present the user with either an opportunity or threat. Some people, upon hearing that they should focus only on the result, will protest that they need to actually work and put their focus on doing things in the right manner. But then there are other people who will find this idea comfortable and they are happy to use any means that are necessary in order to reach that goal.

No matter what your initial reaction is to this thought process, it is important that you learn how to come to the realization that it is always more important to get to the end result that you want, and this needs to come above any of the other considerations that you have.

So, with that in mind, what are some of the ways in which you can put the idea of focusing only on the results, and less on the methods that you use to get there, to practice. We can see this apparent in the professional world. Imagine that you are one of the managers for a company, and you have one employee, in particular, you need to motivate to do more work and to keep up with their job a little bit better.

When you look at this through the view of dark NLP, the only thing that is going to matter is that you are able to get through to your employee and see their motivation increase. This can sometimes conflict with some of the other ideas that are out there about motivation, and some of these will state out how you should talk to the employee and more. But dark NLP isn't going to worry as much about that because it is going to teach the manager that they need to say and do whatever it takes to get the outcome that they want. With dark NLP, the result, and not the journey, is the only thing that is going to matter.

The second attitude to work with when it comes to dark NLP is that you must remember that everything in the world is going to be subjective. Even is two or three people use the same kinds of words in their speech, they could associate different meanings with them in their mind. So, what is this going to mean practically? It is important that you never assume that when someone talks, you automatically know what they mean when they are using a specific word unless there is some evidence of that meaning.

It is also a requirement that you understand how two people could be at the same event or situation but they will have different meanings or different things that they see as important in that event. For example, you could talk to a couple who are about to get married. For the one partner, they are going to be taking the time to participate in a very important religious event. But for the other partner, they may feel that they are just doing something because it is a tradition that is seen as mandatory. Always remember that people are going to work to assign their own meaning to some events.

So, how can dark NLP work with this idea? First, this is going to show that users who are effective with dark NLP are going to be able to influence the way that others around them perceive the situation around them. Let's look at an example of this from management. You are a manager who needs to get the workers to take on some extra hours to ensure that the project gets done by their deadline. In the minds of the workers, it is going to feel that they are being exploited.

But, if the manager has some experience with dark NLP though, they will be able to tie in all of this extra work to the values of the workers. This gives the workers a better chance to take on the hours, and they are less likely to feel guilty or upset about it.

Another thing that this kind of NLP is going to emphasize is the fact that the language people are going to use will not be an absolute representation of what that person is feeling or thinking. You have to spend some time learning about the person and see how they do with their words and how they assign meaning to words, and then you can use this to your advantage.

Use NLP to master your past

There are a lot of different aspects that come with NLP, and we won't have the time to work on all of them in this guidebook. But with some of the core NLP understandings that are covered above will now be filtered down into a series of actionable steps you can take to gain control over the three personal dimensions of time, starting with your past here.

In order to get the most out of this, you will need to be willing to make sure that you are honest with yourself. You must be willing to ace on to all of the choices that you make in your life, and then take the time to analyze them in terms of the results that they are going to generate, and the lessons that you could potentially learn from this. The good news is that this isn't going to be as hard as you may think. Your job here isn't to judge yourself, but you will take a dispassionate look at your lie and identify some of the choices that you made during that time and some of the results that they gave to you.

To get this started, think back to one of the major decisions that you made in your life. It could be an external choice that you made, such as which college you wanted to go with, or something that is more internal, such as a choice to be happier. Whatever it is, you need to jot down a summarized title for the choice, such as choosing a university, being happy, and more.

After you have written down the name of the decisions, you can write down the choices that you were picking through at the time. This also needs to include the decision that you actually chose along with the alternative choices that you didn't go with. Write down as many as you can, but it is best to write down the ones that you were considering during that time. this can then be followed with a summary of what happened with the decision that you made. Did things go as intended? Think through why or why not things worked out, and what you can do to avoid this process.

If you are able to do this process a few times, you may be able to see some patterns emerge in the way that you make and handle decisions. You may find that there are some decision methods that seem to give you the intended outcome, and others that seem to make you get further away from your goals. You can then take a few notes to help you check your future decisions so that you can ensure you are going to make sure that you use the right kind of decision-making process, the one that tends to give you the best results, into the future.

At this point, you should have a nice method that you can use in order to learn from some of the lessons that come up in your past. When you are able to wrap your head around this idea and then you are willing to take some actions on it, you will soon see that there really isn't a need for you to regret the things that happened in your past, because every experience, whether it turned out the way that you wanted or not, is a valuable learning experience.

Making your present better

You will find that dark NLP is not only something that will give you a profound understanding of your past, it is also able to help direct the way that your future is going to head, and it can allow you to live as fully in the present as possible. Dark NLP aims to give tools to help you increase your levels of satisfaction right now, and one way that it is going to do this is by giving you the permission that you need in order to unlock your truest and deepest desires.

There is a method that you can use in order to explore these deepest desires, and they are going to be done through a series of simple and powerful questions. The first thing that you should ask yourself is how you would like to spend a free day if you had no responsibilities and no one else is around to see what you do. The second question is you thinking about how you would spend the lottery win if nobody knew that you had it. And finally, you need to ask yourself what kind of crime you would like to commit if you knew that you were able to get away with it.

When you take the time to give some honest answers to these questions, you can easily see what some of your real desires in life are all about. The power that comes with these questions is that they are going to ask you to think in a way that ensures that the opinion and judgment of others are taken out of the mix. When you take other people out of the mix, you are able to focus on the things that you really want. You may even find that some of the answers that you give are going to surprise you, but other times you may feel inherently at ease with the decisions that you make.

Once you have taken the time to figure out your true desires, you should think about these on a deeper level. For example, you should sit down and think about a situation in which you had uncovered some of your deepest desires, and you found that the desire is to have more money. If this is the case, you can then move into it deeper and think about what money is going to represent for you.

Maybe money is going to represent more freedom. If this is the case for you, then you should combine the deeper representation and the desire into a mantra that you are able to use each day. And if you are able to add in some emotions to these two things, it is going to make that mantra a lot more effective in the long run.

Using NLP to create your new future

And finally, dark NLP is going to provide you with some techniques that will effectively allow you to hack back into your own brain and can make it so that you will brainwash yourself to moving towards your aims, even if you have to do it on autopilot, without the motivation sometimes. To make this work, you first need to tap into the most primal system of reward that exists inside of you. You are going to use a visceral feeling of achievement to help you drive yourself towards this goal.

First, you can stop and do some visualization, picture a time when you have achieved a goal of yours. Think of the raw feelings that came with this win, such as sheer happiness or exhilaration. It is important that you recall this state as much as you can, and spend some time really picturing what it is all about.

You are then going to take some time to picture this great achievement of three goals in your mind that you would like to see accomplished within the next twelve months if possible. Let's say that you want to get your driver's license, you want to finish your degree, and you want to land your first job. With this method, you are going to work to brainwash yourself by linking these three goals with your deepest sense of triumph, the triumph that you felt in the past. This is going to fool the brain into thinking that you already accomplished or experienced your intended outcomes.

To do all of this, you need to keep on with the visualization effort and picture one of the intended outcomes in as clear an image as you can. Spend some time thinking out as many details as you can, and then hold onto this image firmly in your mind. Once that image is there, you can try to make it more vivid and brighter with the eyes of the mind. While that picture is still present, try to summon the good feelings, the ones that you brought up earlier in this exercise. Then try to link this in with the image, until they are connected.

When you are able to do this, you will effectively trick the subconscious into associating a future event with one of the feelings that you went through in the past. The brain won't be able to separate out the two if you were successful with the goal, and this tricks the mind into thinking that the intended outcome already happened.

Because of this, the brain is primed for it to occur, and it is going to seek out to make sure that the goal is going to happen at some point in the future. This can ease the cognitive dissonance that can occur as a result of feeling as if something is in the past, even though it hasn't even had the time to occur in the future for you yet.

By taking the time to picture this image and then recall all of its rich sensory data as much as you can, you are going to take the time to train the mind to accept that goal as something that is actually possible, something that is really within your reach. This can also turn into a powerful source of motivation that you are able to use.

If you are going through this process and there is a time when you feel a bit of resistance in taking action and completing a particular task, then you can come back in and use that visual image that we talked about in this section. When you do this visualization again, you will find that it is essential to take some action to ensure that your vision is going to become a reality.

As you can see, unlike some of the traditional forms of manipulation or psychology, dark NLP allows you to work with all three aspects of time, including the past, the present, and the future. With just a few simple exercises, you are able to use this dark form of NLP to help you get exactly what you want out of life, no matter whether it is a memory of something in the past that you want to improve, if it is something in the present that is going to help you live your life to the fullest or something that you want to change when it comes to the future and reaching your goals overall.

6

Take What You Want, Leave What You Don't

I n this chapter, we are going to take a different approach to dark NLP. We are going to learn more about how to use it in order to influence people, and sometimes even influence yourself. We are now going to take a look at how we can use the dark NLP practices in order to get what we want, no matter how we need to use the techniques on.

The other chapters in this guidebook have been more of a toolkit that you can use in order to carry out what we are going to learn how to do the things that we are going to discuss in this chapter. Having a good understanding of yourself, of your own desires and others can help you to combine all of these into a great technique to get anything that you want out of yourself and out of other people.

The first step to making sure that you are able to get what

you want out of others and out of life is to have the right frame of mind when you get started. You will remember from earlier that one of the core concepts that come with NLP, especially with dark NLP, is that there isn't really a picture of reality that is objective. Instead, we have to really on our own perceptions of it, and these can be really subjective. As a result of this issue, the way in which we frame any given situation has a big impact on how effective you can be with it.

The right frame that you should have when seeking out your own desires in life will be something like "I deserve to get what I want out of life." This may sound really simple, but it can be a bit more difficult than you may originally think. You must not just say the words, you also need to accept and believe them in your own life as well to see the results. If you won't believe these things, then you won't be able to make it happen.

To make sure that you are getting the most out of the life that you already have, you must remember that there really isn't such a thing as scarcity of resources and opportunities. No matter how much people complain about things in our modern world, we live in a time without possibilities that has never been seen before. Anyone is able to get to the sum total of the world's information from the internet, for example, and they can do this from anywhere thanks to wi-fi and their smartphone. This allows you to get all the information that you want on any idea, subject, or skill.

Because of all this abundance that comes with opportunities, you need to realize that you are able to get anything that you want out of life. Once you are able to see how easy it is for you to get what you want, and that this isn't going to deprive anyone else once you do. Other people can use the method that you did in order to see results, they just have to take the first steps.

Morning ritual

One of the foundations of getting what you would like is to build up a series of routines and habits that will enable you to get to those goals as quickly as possible because you are consistent. This chapter is going to focus on providing you with a process that constructs morning and evening routines so that you can stay focused on your path, on your success, and to refine the approach that you use as you go.

The essential purpose of working with a morning routine is to make sure that you go into a state of focus, flow, and peak performance. When you do the same actions in the same order, you will make the transition from sleep to achieving what you want as smooth and as predictable, as possible. Taking this variation out of the mix, the potential for surprises and distraction will be gone, and you are less likely to be drawn away from being productive.

You can make up any kind of schedule that you would like. If you have a small routine that you are used to working with already, you can stick with that a little bit, and then make some changes as you need. A good way to start if you want to make changes to your current routine, or if you want to get a new routine started, you can start to work with a shower in the morning. This can help you to refresh the body and the mind all at once. Adding in a bit of meditation to the process, or repeating your chosen mantras, can make a bit of difference when it comes to how your day goes.

The next stage that you can add into your morning routine is to then move on to prepare some food or beverage that will help you to get set up for the day, and meet your own nutritional values. You could start with some bulletproof coffee, a smoothie, or take on a low carb diet plan in order to see the results that you want. No matter which approach that you have for keeping yourself healthy, make sure that this step isn't missed and that it aligns back with your wider health aims and ideas.

Next, while you are enjoying your food or beverage choices for the day, take some time to go over what goals you want to meet for the day. everyone will have their own method for making this happen. Some may like to write out a list, some may want to write the tasks on a whiteboard or an app. And there are many other methods that you can use. The method that you choose to go with isn't going to be that important, just make sure that you take the time to review your tasks for the day.

The way that you go with the rest of your day is going to depend on your own personal preferences. Some people like to delve into the most challenging part of the day right from the start so that they are able to get it done and over with. Others like to have some more time and maybe they will work in a more nurturing activity, such as reading or doing some mediation. Experiment with it a little bit to see which method is the right one for you.

Evening routines

Once you have mastered the morning routines that you want to work with, it is important to establish some good evening routines as well. Think of your evening and your morning routines as two pieces of the same puzzle, two parts that are going to go together. There are two boundaries to your day, and when you learn how to establish them right, you are going to train the mind to think in terms of achieving a series of aims between the two bookmarks of routines. But what exactly do you want to do when you work on your evening routines.

When setting up a good evening routine for your life, there are going to be two main purposes that you need to focus on. One, you need to learn how to relax the mind and the body so they become ready or rest, and second, you need to take some time to reflect on what has taken place during the day, such as what outcomes you were able to attain. Of course, the order of the routine is going to vary from one person to the next, and when you experiment with the different routines a bit, you will be able to find what is working the best for you. However, a good routine would have a mixture of the processes that we will talk about below.

Many people find that evening is one of the best times to meditate. Typically, when you get to the end of the day, there is a lot of stress and baggage that you took on through the day. The work that you had to get done during the day, the things that went wrong, and your interactions with others will play out in the mind, and in some cases, it can stop us from sleeping and getting the rest that we really need.

To help empty out the mind some more, you can consider adding in some meditation to your evening routine. This is something that won't require a lot of time for you, and it is something that anyone is able to teach themselves how to do. Some of the steps that you can take in order to add some meditation to your routine includes:

1. Get in a position that you find comfortable. Lying down can work, but if you are tired, you may want to sit up so you don't fall asleep.
2. Close your eyes once you are comfortable and take in a series of deep breaths. Try to move your focus over to some of the physical sensations that are now present in the body, rather than on the thoughts and feelings that you have.
3. Start out by sensing the toes, and holding hem tight for a few seconds. Then allow the toes to relax and

notice the feeling of calm that comes with them. Then work the way up the body, doing this with each part as you go, making sure that your focus stays on them.

4. By the time you are to your eyes, you should feel so much more relaxed before. If you have time, you can do some visualization.

5. For this, experience a small ball of white light. Where do you see this ball on the body? Do you see it as glowing or moving? Make the picture as real as you can inside your mind and then allow it to expand and grow. The picture that it is going to get bigger and bigger until this ball of light is able to surround your whole body. Spend a few minutes or so allowing the body to soak up this white light until you get a deep sense of relaxation through all the parts of your body.

Once you have gotten yourself into a state of total and complete relaxation, you can take a look at your day. you could go back through the written list of goals that you had written about in the morning. Which items were you able to achieve, and which ones were too hard, or you just didn't have time for? What was present that made it easier to achieve the goals that you got done?

When you get yourself into the habit of analyzing your goals as a part of your evening routine, you will soon be able to find out which factors are consistently linked back to your failures and which ones are going to be linked back to the triumphs that you had.

You could also choose to incorporate some visualization into your day. you can visualize the following day, and gain a clear image in your mind of how you wish the next day to pan out for you. By taking some time to visualize this, you will prime the mind, making it more likely that this situation is actually going to happen to you.

If you feel up to it, and you feel that it would benefit you a bit, it may be a good idea to keep an in-depth journal. Unlike what we find with a regular journal, there is going to be more specifics with the areas that you need to touch with the dark NLP journal. For example, instead of just going through and focusing on what happened during the day, you should focus more on recording and writing down some of the internal thought processes that you had at the time.

Also, during this activity, spend some time pondering why you have arrived at a specific subjective understanding of the day, or why another meaning may not be the best fit for you, at least at this time. When you focus on doing this, you will soon gain a better understanding of your own thought processes and the way that your own mind is going to work. Over time, you will see patterns and can use this information in order to model some of your own peak states, allowing you to enter into them on a more consistent basis.

Input = output

One of the core principles of NLP questions if the influence we take in have a direct influence on the output, or what we get out of life. It is our duty, and party our responsibility, to ourselves, that we only allow the right kinds of influences into our lives at all times. While the traditional view that comes with NLP could state that these inputs should be any that will promote wellbeing and health, our more ruthless version of NLP, the dark NLP, is going to teach us that any type of input that allows us to go after our desires is one that we should allow into our lives.

It is worth our time to go after an input that is going to serve our aims in a direct manner, no matter the morality of the input. For example, if you are in the world of business, you may search for some time before coming across a book that is going to offer you the techniques and tools that you need to become a bit more effective with what you are doing. Once you read it a little further, you may discover the techniques will include several that go against what is seen as social norms.

If you went and saw these techniques and decided to reject the book right then and there, you would not be thinking along the ideas of dark NLP. Your only concern with this would be deciding whether the book is going to offer you any inputs that will help you reach your aims, regardless of how moral they are, if you were using dark NLP.

One of the key tests to consider when it comes to deciding on input is whether it is going to disempower you or empower you and whether it teaches you how to be passive or active. This is going to stem back to the earlier exploration of the idea that, in any given situation, one party is going to be the prey and one is going to be the predator. Make sure that you are being proactive in the choices that you make to ensure you become the predator in all situations, and that you actually reach what you are striving for.

Aim high without limits

The last thing that we are going to explore in this chapter is that you should aim high, and not limit yourself. One of the big mistakes that people are going to make in the world of dark NLP is that they will think too small. Too many people aim for changes that are relatively minor, rather than going for the bold and big changes that dark NLP is able to provide to you.

A big reason that a lot of people are going to aim their sights so low is that they are afraid of failing. Many of us worry that we are not that good, that we aren't good enough to actually achieve the things that we aim for. And so we will aim low in order to make sure that we are protected from the pain of failure. But if you aim this low, you are going to end up selling yourself short, and you will really miss out on all the cool and wonderful things that you are able to do.

If you have taken the time to internalize some of the lessons that we have looked at in this book, you will learn that there isn't something like a failure. Rather there is feedback instead. You should not hold yourself back from dreaming in a big manner and aiming for some big achievements in your life. If you do not get there the first time, this doesn't mean that you have failed. You just learned a valuable lesson to help you progress the next time that you attempt your goals.

Another reason to set some really big goals for yourself is that even if you do end up falling short a bit, you still worked hard and pushed your limits. When you manage to make yourself accept this logical reason to set some of the bigger goals, you will start to feel more comfortable in doing so. And as you push your limits and try to get more and more done, you will be amazed at all of the cool things that you can do.

7

You Have the Advantage, Learn How to Exploit That

With any new thing that you are trying to do and the techniques that you are going to learn from that, there is going to be a kind of learning curve along the way. you will be able to look at some insight into some of the typical stages of progress that occur when someone is learning dark NLP for the first time. Each of the different stages of progress will clearly be described out to you, and then you will have the advice that is needed in order to progress to the ultimate aim of dark NLP, which is to become a constant predator.

To start with is the first stage of dark NLP. This first stage is often known as a tentative form of exploration. During this stage, someone who has heard about the dark NLP and some of the unique ways that it is able to change your perspective on life and the world will begin to consider its ideas, and then can weigh these new ideas against some of their own perceptions of the world.

When you reach to this point, it is possible for the person not to agree with the ideas of dark NLP, they may agree with some of the parts but not all of them, or they may decide that they agree completely with the ideas that come with dark NLP. These individuals are merely judging them in light of the experience that they personally have. To help the individual go beyond this kind of phase, it is advised that you actively seek to apply your understanding of dark NLP to the world around you.

After you have spent a little bit of time looking at dark NLP and some of the basics that come with it, and you have had some time to see whether the ideas are a good match with your own personally views of reality, you may agree that there is at least the potential of dark NLP to be useful. This is the stage of the process that is often known as cautious acceptance. It is during this time that you will start using the lens of dark NLP, but it still takes some conscious effort to look at the world in that manner. You may even start to question your own understanding of morality when you are in this part.

The next thing that you want to work on is figuring out how to push beyond the cautious acceptance. You are able to do this by making a conscious effort to put some of the techniques of dark NLP to the motion. You will want to specifically pay attention to any of the techniques that are related to influencing yourself, as well as others, as fast as you can. You will find that through more experience and practice, and for seeing personal success, using a technique, you will find that it is easier to accept these techniques in your life.

Following the cautious acceptance that we talked about above, you will then need to progress to a new level of using dark NLP that is going to be known as casual competence. When you are at this stage, you will stop having to put in so much effort to use the dark NLP techniques. You will start to naturally think in terms of dark NLP concepts, and over time, it is going to require progressively less effort on your part. You may even find that you are able to use the ideas of dark NLP to take control over your own life and to make sure that you are able to influence others near you, without even having to think about it.

The biggest distinction that comes with this is that once you reach this stage, it is going to show that you are to a new level of progress. You will know it has happened when you realize that you have gained some influence over others, and when you realize this, there isn't a level of guilt that comes with it.

To make sure that you are able to get the most out of this stage, it is important to begin to put it into practice, and to make sure that you track down the patterns that you see with your success. You may find that at this stage of your progress, you are going to benefit from keeping a journal so that you are able to keep track of the different routines that you do, and what happens to work well for your success. You stand the best chance of moving past this particular stage if you can learn how to identify the difference between those times when you are successful, and the times you are not.

We can then move on to the level that is beyond casual competence. These are all going to involve a good mastery of Dark NLP, one that can take a long time to reach and succeed at. There are no longer so many levels that are distinct when it comes to progress as there are gradual degrees of improvement. Signs that someone has gotten to this stage of dark NLP is going to include many things such as the ability to read the power balance no matter what situation you are in, the ability to mirror the other person without even thinking about it, and even how to influence the other person with some deep and artificial rapport, without all the effort.

The mastery that you have of dark NLP is going to be reliant on how willing you are to absorb some of the concepts and techniques that are described in this guidebook. To make this happen, you need to be willing and able to take some big actions in your life to get the right influence with dark NLP. You also need to be willing to figure out what patterns are going to lead you to success, and then use this to reach the next level of your mastery in the shortest space of time as possible.

As you are looking through your feelings and your emotions, you will come to a part that your mind is going to automatically think in terms of the concepts that are important to dark NLP. Once this happens, you will be able to interact with someone in a way that is going to force some rapport with them before exploiting them for your own needs. This means that you have gotten to the ultimate goal that comes with dark NLP, which means that you are now a constant predator.

A personal SWOT

The next thing that we need to take a look at here is known as a personal SWOT. This is an acronym that is going to talk about strengths, weaknesses, opportunities, and threats. This is a tool that a lot of different businesses like to work with to help them come up with marketing campaigns and to ensure that they are going to beat out the competition. But you can create one for your own use that is going to provide insight into the different positive and negative aspects of a person.

So, how do you go through this and make it work for yourself? The first thing that you should ask yourself is to figure out what your main strengths are, and your main weaknesses. You may want to go through and jot down a list of the things that you see as strengths and weaknesses. The order doesn't matter here, you just want to make sure that it is as complete as possible.

After you have had some time to write down all of the different aspects that fit into these two categories that you can, you can then narrow them down. This analysis is going to take way too long if you have to sort through twenty or more things for example. Pick out the top five things that you can begin to work on and then rank them. This gives you a look at the view of your major weaknesses and strengths and we can work from there.

After you take some time to find your strengths and weaknesses, which are basically the view that you have with your inner self at the time, then it is important to analyze the range of possible opportunities that are going to exist inside your life right now, and any threats that could cause a disruption to the current way of life that you have.

Now, one of the things that you need to remember about here is that your weaknesses are not something that should be seen in a negative light here. Your weaknesses here are areas where there is a lot of chances for you to improve things. Let's say that three of the personal weaknesses that you want to focus on will include bad presentation skills, limited social life, and a low amount of confidence when you speak out in public. Instead of looking at these like weaknesses, you can look at them more like a puzzle that you need to spend some time-solving. Once you are able to solve the puzzle and get all of the pieces to work together, you will be able to solve those weaknesses and get them to work for you.

You are able to use the information that you get in the SWOT to work with several of the techniques of dark NLP, such as choosing your habits, influencing others, and envisioning your future.

Breaking the rapport

Up to this point, we have spent a lot of time talking about the different ways that you can build up some rapport with the other person, making sure that they are soft to your influence. Now we need to take a moment to learn the best way to break this rapport, and then build it back up over a period of time.

Before you are able to take control over another person by breaking the rapport, it is important that you come up with a solid level of rapport. This is going to be achieved through the physical and linguistic mirroring techniques that we talked about earlier on. You then need to make sure that you reach the stage o influence where you are able to lead the body language of the other person you are interacting with. Once you have reached this level, then you are ready to begin the process of breaking the rapport in a tactical manner.

To break the rapport with the other person, it is time to stop mirroring them. Stop using the markers for linguistics that you found earlier. Switch over to a brusque and negative tone of voice and do anything that is going to seem like you are trying to get away from the rapport. You will know that this is successful because the other person in the conversation is going to start acting like they are dejected or confused.

When you do break out of this deep rapport that you had done and worked so hard on earlier, there are going to be two effects that happen right away with them. First, the other person is going to feel like there was some kind of loss that happened because all of the good emotions that you sent their way will be gone. Second, you are going to trigger the natural inclination of the other person to chase after and seek your validation in order to fill up the void of your approval.

Of course, once you are successful at breaking the rapport with the other person, you do still allow them a chance to regain the rapport again. The timing of this is going to need to be strategic in the way that you are able to reward the desired behavior or statement of the other person before you give in. for example, if the other person is trying to regain the rapport with you and they touch you, and you want them to repeat this, you would then reconnect rapport with them at that time. they would make the link of good feelings of the rapport with this behavior and repeat it in the future.

You will find that breaking the rapport that you have built up with the other person can be a really powerful tool, and it is one that you should use in a sparing manner. It is often best to deploy it to make sure that there is sometimes the element of chase and tension in the interaction and to help with the emotional progress that you are building. It is possible to build and break the rapport a few times in the same communication but do be careful about overdoing it. The more that you do this, the harder it is going to be to rebuild that deep rapport and if you push it too much, then you are going to make it so that the person isn't even interested in you anymore.

8

Hypnotic Seduction and How It Works

I n this chapter, we are going to take some time to look at how some of the principles that come with dark NLP can be used to help you be more successful with romantic endeavors. No matter what romantic goals that you have, this chapter is still going to provide you with a personal blueprint that will make it easier to achieve them and get the results that you want.

The first thing that has to happen if you would like to use the ideas of dark NLP in a romantic way is to start eliminating some of the limiting beliefs you may have had in the past about this subject. There are a few limiting beliefs that often keep showing up, and they are going to make it harder for you to have the romantic seduction that you are looking for.

The most common of these limiting beliefs is that if you use the ideas of dark NLP to seduce someone, it is somehow seen as wrong or immoral. There are two sources for this particular limiting belief. The first is that the view of seduction needs to happen in a particular way, and the second issue is that there is really a big misunderstanding of exactly what the dark NLP seduction is going to entail.

We often believe that seduction needs to look a certain way because we have seen it in that manner through books and movies, rather than experiencing it firsthand. This can make us believe that things that make the best move scenes are going to be the ones that represent the process of one person becoming attracted to another. And if there is anything that goes against this in our lives, or in the lives of others, then it is going to mean that we reject it when something goes against our conceptions.

There are also those who are against the idea of the hypnotic seduction because they think that it takes the choice away from the other person, and they think that this kind of seduction is going to force the target into doing something that they don't want to do. However, this is not the truth.

With hypnotic seduction, we are basically learning how to connect better with someone, to connect with them on a deeper level than we could with other techniques, and we learn how to trigger some good emotions when the other person thinks about you. The target is going to have all of the freedom of choice that they want, and they will not be forced into the situation. But you are just using your own influence your chances by your ability to give the other person a good experience and connect with you far faster than what you can with some of the other techniques.

And then there is the issue that some people are going to be really worried that they are not able to understand, or that they won't be able to actually use, some of the techniques that are needed to use the dark NLP for romantic things. This objection sounds logical, but it is going to be used as a type of mask of something deeper, such as having a fear of connecting to some of the other people in your life, or some other personal insecurity. You can overcome these and learn how to use dark NLP to help you to do well with personal romance, but you have to take the steps first to make this happen.

The theory of romantic seduction

There are going to be a few foundations that are going to underpin what we will talk about in the remainder of this chapter. These ideas are going to take some time to explain why some of the principles of dark NLP can be so effective, especially when compared to other techniques when it comes to seducing others. This section can be more about why that comes behind the use of hypnotic seduction, and we can look at the how in a little bit.

The first idea which is key to your understanding of

hypnotic seduction is the idea that we inherently seek out others they feel comfortable secure around. They want to make sure that they get in a relationship with someone who is going to make them feel good and secure as much as possible. This is a process that is often going to happen over a longer period of time, as the couple, or two people, start to do a lot of different shared activities together to get to know one another a little bitter.

But when you bring in some of the principles that come with dark NLP, you are able to speed up this process, and this sense of shared experience and it allows people to connect quicker than they would be able to do in the traditional methods of seduction.

The second main idea that can come with dark NLP in your seduction efforts is that people are going to try and find others who will share in the same values that they do. This can be kind of hit and miss in some cases, and it is going to take some time since the deepest values that someone has can take some time to show up. But when we bring out some of the ideas that come with dark NLP, you are able to bring out some of those deeper values much faster than before.

From there, you need to come to the understanding that people are usually not as in control over their own actions as they think. When you are able to read some of their actions, and some of their choices in language, you are able to really influence them on a deeper level. This is usually going to be a case of presenting the strongest reality relative to the one you would like to seduce and influence in order to get the results that you want.

How to create the hypnotic mood

The first thing that we need to look at for this kind of seduction is making sure that we are able to create the right mood. There are going to be a few factors that will contribute to what makes the perfect mood for seduction with dark NLP. In most cases, there shouldn't be any background noise that is going to distract the target from the conversation that is going on right now. However, you may want to add in a bit of music or something so that the silences aren't going to become so awkward between you and your target.

After you make sure that the levels of noise in the background are right where you want them, it is important to make sure that you end up in some kind of environment where you are unlikely to get disturbed. This doesn't mean that you can't go out in public and do the interaction. These techniques do just fine when you are out and about in public. It is even possible to carry some of these in louder areas, such as a nightclub. But the key here is that even if other people are around you, you want to make sure that you are choosing a location where you minimize other people coming into the conversation and interrupting you.

The surroundings that you use are going to be informal and

relaxed to see the best results. This ensures that both you and the target you are working with are as comfortable as possible and that you can both work to communicate as deeply with one another as possible. If you pick out an atmosphere that feels too formal or makes one or the other of you feel too uncomfortable, then it is going to make it almost impossible for the romance or intimacy that you want to create to even occur.

You can also pick out an area where you can be close enough for physical contact if needed. This doesn't mean that things like kissing are going to automatically happen. But it is possible. If you pick out a location, make sure that some of this physical contact can happen without judgment from others.

Seductive anchoring

The anchoring tactic is going to come into play for this part of the process. This means that seductive anchoring is going to involve helping the target to feel deep feelings of positive emotion. They then have these feelings tied right back to you. What this does is that when the target is near you, if you used anchoring in the proper manner, they are going to have a positive emotion about this, and it can even become a valuable part of their lives as well.

To get started with the seductive anchoring, you must make sure that the frame that is between yourself and the other target is romantic. Both you and the target need to be aware that the time you are spending together is going to signify something that is more important and more serious than just being friends. Otherwise, all of the efforts that you are going to work with when it comes to anchoring will result in a deepening of friendship connections, rather than the romance that you are looking for.

When you are ready to do some romantic interactions with the other person, you want to make sure that you are their guide to going into a state of positive emotions that are strong. One way for you to do this is to guide the other person into asking lots of questions and then asking the other person to recall the memories that they have from childhood that are their fondest. You want to make sure that they spend some time talking on the topic, and that they share some of the details as they can. Every time that you ask a question that is going to bring out a positive feeling with the other person, you can do a subtle gesture, one that you can continually repeat without too much attention, such as touching on your wrist.

When you go through and repeat this physical gesture while invoking a positive emotion in the target, you are basically going to link the physical stimulus with the emotion that is in the mind of the person. After you repeat this enough times in front of the other person, you can then use this to your advantage to invoke that positive feeling in the person any time that you would like, simply by using that physical cue to help you out.

Another way that you are able to work with seductive anchoring is as a way of ensuring that the target that you are spending your time with is feeling comfortable and good when they are around you. You must have some good intentions around them though to make sure that this is going to work for your needs. When you are comfortable and having a good time, and you really want them to have the same, they are more likely to feel good around you each time that you get together, and it is easier to seduce them into liking you as well.

You may find that seductive anchoring will be best used when you are trying to enhance an existing romantic interaction, rather than using it as the basis for the relationship. There are some people who will start to realize the power of the technique, and then they start to make the mistake of thinking it is a form the foundation of their romantic encounter. But this is a big mistake.

For the seduction with dark NLP to work, there has to already be something of substance between you and your target. There should be genuine chemistry or at least the appearance of it. Seductive anchoring can really help to enhance the connection that is already present between people, but it is not going to be able to create a brand new one.

Us vs. Them technique

One of the actionable steps that you are able to work with is where you will create a sense of connection and intimacy during the course of seduction. This is a technique that is going to work to create a shortcut to feel that they are going to share a secret with you or a special kind of relationship with someone. These connections usually don't happen until a long period of time has happened, but with the dark NLP techniques, you can make this happen in no time at all.

One of the reasons that the long term friendships feel so special and important to us is because we are going to set up a shared set of references, including some inside jokes, and even a secret language, with the people you are trying to seduce. Dark NLP is going to offer you a few different techniques that you can use to ensure this kind of thing is going to happen in a short amount of time.

To make this happen, you should first start out with some inside jokes with whomever you are working to seduce. This could be coming up with a silly kind of nickname that they like and that only you can call them. You can come up with a word for something that happens, or something else that is special and only between the two of you.

Any time that it is possible, you should use a technique that is known as callback humor to help with the us vs. them approach. Once you have come up with a few unique sayings and names that show how you and hat other person have a special connection. By recalling these phrases that you share, you are going to create a special sense of shared history and humor that is going to make the other person feel more comfortable around you than they would around someone else in a similar amount of time.

You can really deepen the sense of us vs. them when you take some time to emphasize the commonalities that show up between yourself and the other person you would like to become romantic with. For example, if you go out with someone and order the same drink as them while you are out, you can use this small detail in order to come up with a basis for a funny story about how you both must have great taste since you both ordered that drink.

Don't underestimate this technique. Even things that seem minor and unimportant can be enough for a basis to make unique and quirky connections. You should always be aware of which connections your person of interest is going to respond to the best and to make sure that you get a positive response, and then give up the ones that aren't getting the positive reception.

The use of embedded stories

Another method that you can use is known as embedded stories. This is a way that you can share some deep and meaningful values with someone you would like to pursue in a romantic manner. The concept that comes with these embedded stories is that it comes with the idea of tribe theory. This is a theory that states when seeking out a romantic partner, people are going to look for a partner who is in the same social tribe as themselves, is in a superior tribe to theirs, or is in a tribe that is different, but equal, to the one that the person wants to experience.

This theory, when you use it with dark NLP, is going to state that people are going to have different types of values depending on the tribe that they are in. For example, the values of their own tribe will be those hat the person is going to hold for their own, and are in conjunction with the general social expectations for someone in their standing. And then the values that are found in a tribe they consider as superior to their own are ones that this person holds as values to aspire to. And then the value of any tribes they find interesting, but they will feel is too taboo to enter because of some social pressure.

The first step that we need to follow when it comes to using the theory of tribes is to figure out which tribe you will work to portray yourself as being inside. The method of this is going to be simple. If you genuinely share a lot in common with the person you want to seduce, it is often best if you are able to get yourself to appear like you are in the same tribe as them. But if there are things in place that put you into a higher standing, such as more educated or some other reason, then it is best to portray yourself as being in a tribe that is superior.

Once you have settled with a tribal identity that you will convey during the course of the seduction with the other person, you will then need to figure out the values that you are going to showcase, the ones that will show the other person which tribe you are in.

So, if you have decided to portray yourself as coming from a higher up tribe, which values do you think the object of your affection thinks goes with that tribe with that person. Having a good understanding of the values that you would like to convey to the other person is going to be so important when you try to embed them into the stories that you talk about.

The main purpose of having a good and effective embedded story is to convey certain compatibility with the other person, while still trying to occupy up space in their logical mind by telling a story that is engaging. The aspects that will convey the value are going to be hidden, and will not be the primary focus of the story. Instead, these facts are going to be woven in through the use of body language, and other forms of communication as well.

Let's take a look at some of the examples that you are able to use that go along with this idea as well. Imagine that you have met someone and you have decided that you want to show off hat you come from the same kind of tribe as that person. And you have taken some time to identify that one of the values of this tribe was reliability.

When you are talking to that other person, you may slip in a story. On the surface, this story seems to be about at rip that you took while on vacation. Make sure that the story is interesting enough that it is going to hold onto the attention of your target, but the language needs to be able to subtly relate some phrases of reliability into it, such as "I never let people down" "I chose them because they offer a reliable service" and so on.

The benefits of going through and telling one of these embedded stories is that it is going to allow you to associate a great type of value to yourself, one that the logical mind of the other person is not going to question. Because you took the time to distract them with the linear story, they are going to actually value the allusions at a deeper level. This can make it easier for you to influence how the other person perceives you. By choosing the right value, and going with the one that provides you with a great chance of seducing that person, and you are going to get a ton more out of what appears to be a simple conversation than what others can get with small talk.

Using some signature touches and gestures

Some of the speakers who are the most known throughout history are the ones who are known for making certain motions or gestures when they speak. For you to make sure that the other person finds you as charismatic as possible, you should make sure to stick with some specific motions when you speak. It is important that the gestures aren't just random though. You need to make sure that they go along with the kind of tone that you are using with your communication.

For example, if you are talking about the other person opening up, then you may find that working with an open gesture is going to help to emphasize the point that you are trying to use. This is going to ensure that your words and your actions are aligned together well.

If you use these signature motions sparingly, and you are able to use them on a consistent basis to coincide with a certain function of your speech, then you will find that the other person sees you as a more memorable and charismatic, and they are more likely to remember you in the future. Remember, that while words are important, only a small part of the meaning that we are able to convey to someone is going to be associated with our words. Much more of it is going to be through other aspects such as body language and tone.

What this means is that when we use our body language to our own advantage, and we make sure that we are using consistent motions and gestures, you will be able to condition the person we are interacting with to respond to us consistently when triggered by the gesture.

When you feel that you have gained a good level of comfort and connection with the other person, it is then a sign that you can start to explore some of the subtle ways that actually touching the other person can do. You may find that once you are able to get the other person to start laughing, and you start to touch them gently on the arm, they are going to start associate this emotion with the touch, and therefore, back to you.

When you are using a technique like touch, you need to be careful about using them too much. These techniques are going to work so well because they are going to work right under the radar, and they are something that is not understood on a conscious basis. Because of this, they won't be able to trigger the usual rational thought processes or the mechanisms that are in place for defense, when you are interacting them. If you have been overusing it, especially with touches, then people will start to register what you are doing, and their guard is going to go up right away.

9

Some of the Masters of NLP, and How You Can Learn From Them

There are a lot of masters when it comes to working with NLP. And there is a lot that we are able to learn from them. Let's take a look at some of the people who have helped to influence the world of NLP, and some of the things that we can learn from them.

Ross Jeffries

Ross Jeffries is one of the most divisive and notorious names when it comes to the world of NLP. He is known for taking some of the concepts that come with NLP and then applying them in a way to see how they influence seduction. Jeffries is said to actually be the basis for several characters from Hollywood who would exhibit behaviors of self-assurance and being cocky. And many people loathe him because he used a lot of shock value techniques in marketing in order to draw some unneeded negative attention to NLP.

Jeffries is sometimes remembered for having some high profile disagreements that he ended up having with some of his former students. A theme that was found with most of these is that Jeffries felt that the other person was treating him unfairly. In the book of seduction known as The Game, the author detailed how Jeffries would often become bitter if there was another teacher who showed some conflicts to understanding seduction the way that Jeffries did.

One of the biggest contributions that Ross Jeffries brought to us and to the world of NLP is his ability to take the principles that we have been talking about in NLP and refined them for a specific purpose. While there had been many users of NLP who were aware of the fact that they could use NLP for romantic reasons, Jeffries was the first to come up with a system of doing this.

Jeffries was also one of the first to tap into the potential of marketing NLP in a way that suggested that those who decided to use it would almost have a kind of superpower. He was able to suggest that one someone purchased one of the products he sold or went to one of his seminars, they would be able to have a godlike level of control over anyone they wanted. While it is true that the use of NLP can really enhance how much influence you can have over someone else, Jeffries made it seem like even more than that.

Jeffries also brought in a lot of new terms and jargon that could be used with the idea of NLP. Before this, a lot of the principles and techniques that were used with this were not named, and there could be some confusion amongst those who were working with this method. However, Jeffries was able to contribute to some technical jargon that helped refer to the various concepts that came with NLP.

Tony Robbins

The next person to take a look at is Tony Robbins. Robbins is one of the most recognizable teachers of self-improvement and motivation throughout the world. And he is known for all of the seminars and products that people can use in order to help people take control of their lives and see the results and outcomes that they have always wanted.

Since he started off with his earliest book, we did mention a bit about the power of NLP and how it could help you to achieve some fast results. In fact, Robbins even spent some time advocating about NLP and how it could help people get what they wanted out of life, how it could help to motivate themselves to take action, and to make sure that they reach the end result that they want.

Robbin's has a unique take when it comes to NLP, and it included the ability to combine it together with some of the other concepts for reaching your goals in order to enhance how strong it is. for example, Robbins found that it was possible to combine together the ideas of NLP visualizations with methods that were drawn from literature related to goal setting and time management. This was done with the goal of setting up a system so that others had a really strong system, one that was stronger than what the individuals could do with the individual components of the system on its own.

In addition, Robbins took some time to directly link the benefits of using NLP back to some of the teachings and techniques that he used for his own. Often people are going to be turned off from the ideas and concepts of NLP because they worry that it is going to be something that is used for evil. But Robbins made a stance because he was able to convince people that it was fine to use NLP, and showed a lot of ways that NLP was able to improve their lives with these concepts.

Robbins was able to build up some good trust in himself, and back to his methods at the same time because he was able to present them with an impressive track record. No matter where he was on the career path, Robbins was able to refer back to some of the past achievements that he had reached as a way to show that his techniques and concepts were credible. And since he was one of the most prominent teachers that were considered mainstream, he was able to really form that connection when it comes to understanding what our values are and then tying them into our everyday activities to give them more meaning.

Derren Brown

Derren Brown is an entertainer who was able to use a blend of psychology and NLP in order to achieve a lot of influence over those who he encountered over the years. In many ways, the methods that Brown used were close to what we are talking about here with dark NLP. Because of this, Brown is going to combine together the insights to some of the unknown aspects of the human psyche with the concepts and tactics that come with NLP in order to get some results that tended to work.

One of the defining features that come with Brown is that he had the ability to make other people do things and carry out other types of behavior that to the outsider seemed completely amazing. Occasionally, one of the books or television specials that Brown provided would offer a rare insight into some of the ideas and techniques that he would use to make this happen. What most of his abilities seem to have in common is that they are used in order to manipulate the nuances of human behavior to act in a certain manner.

One reason that we are taking a look at Brown is that he was an entertainer who was able to take just a single principle from NLP and then turned it into an entertaining and amazing visual spectacle. For example, Brown would be able to show off the power of an embedded order or a command and could do this, and some of the tactics that we talked about in this guidebook, in order to get those in his audience to behave and do things that were seen as extraordinary.

In one instance, Brown was filmed visiting a series of shops in NYC. He was there using blank pieces of paper as a banknote. When he started to talk with the shop worker, Brown was able to keep the logical mind occupied by telling some mundane story to them. When it was time for Brown to pay, Brown would issue the command, "Take it, it's fine" within the confines of his story.

For example, he may have had a story set up about how reluctant he was to catch the subway on time. But because he was able to put in that embedded order, he was then able to influence the worker at the shop to take the piece of paper, even though it was blank.

There were other things that Brown was able to do in order to combine stage magic, the principles that come with showmanship, and NLP. He often takes an idea from NLP, such as its techniques of helping people have some really strong visualizations that are based on sensory data. Brown was able to apply this kind of idea when he had a volunteer perceive their own senses as if they were actually a wooden dummy.

Now, this may have looked pretty amazing to those who were watching. But all that Brown had to do in order to get the other person to carry out his desires was to use some of the techniques that came with NLP. He simply changed it around a bit in order to really captivate the audience at the same time.

As you can see, there are a lot of different ways that NLP

can be used. And the topics that we are discussing in this guidebook are not meant to just be theories and things to talk about. With the examples above, you will find that the thoughts of NLP can be used for a variety of reasons, to ensure that you are able to have the influence over others that you are looking for, without having to force them to act in this manner.

10

Inaction is the same as Death

Now that you have gone through the other chapters of this guidebook, you should now have a complete picture of how dark NLP works, and some of the immense power that it has to affect and change up all of the aspects and areas of your life. You know more about how to take control over yourself first, and with that knowledge, you are able to extend your influence out to the others who are around you.

Now that you know all of this information, it is time to choose how you want to interact. Many people are interested in getting started with dark NLP, and they are worried about where to go from there. They may decide to start learning a bit about NLP, and then get stuck because they aren't sure what steps to take next. Remember, when it comes to dark NLP, doing nothing is the same as killing off your dreams. If you really want to reach your goals and your desires in life, you have to always be moving, always in action. And once that happens, amazing things are going to change in your life.

Getting from the starting line is going to be the hardest.

Many people, when they are trying to grasp the power of Dark NLP for the first time, will feel a little paralyzed with all of the information. They start to realize some of the richness that can come with this power, and this can leave them feeling intimidated and unsure of what they should do to deal with this new freedom.

Once you learn about dark NLP, remember that the hardest part of the journey is going to be the first step. When you start to get going, you will start to build up some momentum, which is going to carry you forward on the journey. But beginning, and getting past that starting line, is the hardest part because you have no momentum to get you going. It is up to you to use some of the ideas and the tools that we have been talking about in this guidebook to help you take the right actions.

The best way for you to get started here is to think of the one small step, even the easiest step, which you can take in order to make a little bit of progress in all the major areas of your life. For example, maybe you want to get your health in line. to do this, you know that you need to eat right, join a gym, and start to work out on a regular basis. When you look at it this way, it all seems like a big task. But taking the first step, such as finding the prices of gyms in your area, can help you to get started, and provides you with the motivation that you need to keep going and get healthy.

Dream big

There are many things in life that will come up and make it so that you are held back, and the scope of your ambition will be put on hold as well. Ironically, there are very few limitations are as damaging to you like the ones that you try to place on yourself.

Don't ever let the ways that you will use this book, and the information that is inside of it, be held back by issues like doubt or a lack of self-belief. Try to believe and understand that there are really no limits to the potential that you can reach. There are so many ordinary people who are able to make a difference and achieve extraordinary things all of the time. Since they believe in themselves, they will continue to do this for the long term.

Live by the code that you invented

The ideas and the techniques that we talk about in this guidebook are at some point going to raise up some different ethical considerations and questions that you need to figure out. While you are reading through some of the sections, you may have felt a level of discomfort at different points. You may be worried about how you would be able to influence someone else, and whether you would be performing actions that were considered ethical or not based on some of the social norms that you have to deal with today.

However, you will find that the parts that you respond to in a negative or uncomfortable manner may not be the same that other people run into issues. Some people are going to find that they are the most uncomfortable about dreaming in a big manner and having to set some big goals for their own lives. Other people will find that their level of discomfort is going to come from exerting influence over others.

The thing to remember for this is that instead of following a code of ethics that match up with society, you should devise your own code of ethics. Often the code of ethics that society provides to you is going to hold you back and will make it difficult for you to reach the goals that you have set for yourself. And this will make it difficult for you to get the things that you want out of life.

But when you take the time to devise your own code of ethics, you are able to decide what you are willing to do, and what you aren't willing to do. Remember that we talked a bit earlier about how morality is going to be different for everyone. And for some individuals and rules of thought with dark NLP, nothing is seen as morally wrong as long as it helps you to reach your end goals.

You don't have to go through and take it this far. It is fine to have some ethics in place, and some limits that you aren't willing to cross, but that doesn't mean that your ethics and your limits have to be the same as what society puts in place. You can develop some of your own and work from there.

To do this, find out the exact way that you feel about the different concepts and the different tactics that we talked about in this guidebook, and see where your discomfort level is going to rest. Remember, you are able to go through and refine and adapt your code of ethics at any time during the journey. But even if you do make some changes to it later, always make sure that you have your own code of ethics in place all of the time. Without this code of ethics in place, you will have no idea about what you find acceptable, and what is not.

No matter what you decide your code of ethics is about, you should feel that dark NLP is intended to be liberating and empowering. You should be able to use it in a guilt-free manner. This ensures that you are able to enjoy the results that you get, and the act that you reach your goals, with the help of NLP.

Learn how to shape the world the way that you see fit

One of the core messages that you should take away from learning dark NLP, and that we have been talking about in this guidebook, is that it allows you to be the one in the driver's seat. You no longer need to sit back and be passive or accept what life has handed to you. With these techniques, you are able to figure out the different ways that people think, and why they do certain things, and then use this information to your own advantage.

The best thing about all of this power is that you are then able to exert influence on the world and everyone around you. You can use the concepts that we discuss in this guide-book to lead people, and to lead various situations, to make sure that you reach your end goals, and get the things that you want. For example, if you believe that it is better if people start showing more of a certain value or behavior, dark NLP will be able to help you push others in that direction.

To make sure that you are able to fulfill the potential of all this influence, you must have a clear idea of what you would like to achieve along the way. having an overall strategy or approach to life will make sure that you stay consistent, that you come up with decisions that are based on your princi-ples, and making a decision that will have an impact on the world around you that is certain to make you happy.

The goal and the role of this book is not to take the time to judge the vision that you have in mind. That is up to you. Whatever you choose to make the world into is up to your discretion. You owe it to yourself to come up with a vision that is entirely yours, one that doesn't have a lot of external influences with it. If you let others start to control the vision that you have for your life, you are going to lose and won't get the outcome that you want.

So, the last question that you need to ask yourself here is what you would like out of life? No matter what your goals are, or what you would like out of life, you are now out of excuses to not get to work and make it a reality. Now that you know, every second count. And each second that you are not getting out there and taking the right actions to make this a reality is a second that is wasted. When you have the powerful knowledge that comes with NLP, why not use it to your advantage.

11

Easy Techniques to Use with NLP

This guidebook has taken a lot of time to talk about dark NLP and how it is able to help you make a change in the world, and get more of the things that you want out of life. No matter what your personal code of ethics is like, you will find that dark NLP can be used in a way that helps to benefit yourself and helps you to reach your goals. Now it is time to take a look at some of the different NLP techniques that you can use in order to help make a major transformation in your own life and to ensure that you are able to get other people to react in the way that you want.

Dissociation

. . .

The first thing that we are going to take a look at is a process that is known as dissociation. Have you ever entered into a certain situation and just had a really bad feeling about it right from the start? Or maybe there are certain situations where you are going to start feeling sad or down each time that you experience it. Or you may have some situations at work that are going to make you pretty nervous, such as a situation where you need to speak publicly.

These situations show the whole range of emotions that you can have, and often they are going to seem like things that you have to deal with, ones that are automatic, and unstoppable. But you will find that using the techniques from dark NLP, and using dissociation, you will be able to turn these feelings away and not allow them to bother you any longer. Some of the ways that you can make this happen includes:

1. Identify the emotion that you want to spend some time on, the one that you want to target and get rid of. This can be any kind of emotion that you want such as disliking the situation, discomfort, rage, and fear.

2. Once you have picked out the feeling that you want to work with, you can imagine that you have the ability to float out of your body, and then look back at yourself. This gives you a chance to encounter

the whole situation from a different perspective, of that of the observer.

3. Once you take yourself out of the situation and just get to watch what is going on, rather than needing to actively participate in it, you will find that your own personal feelings about that particular situation will start to change.

4. You may find that you don't feel as shy, that the public speaking isn't as big of a deal as you had thought, or maybe you are now able to talk to that person you liked, the one who made you feel nervous in the beginning.

5. To get an added boost to this, you can first imagine that you are able to float out of your body looking at yourself, and then you can float out of this body again so that you can look at yourself looking at yourself. This is a process that is known as double dissociation and it can ensure that you are really removed from the situation and that all of the negative emotions that come with many minor situations are long gone so that you are better able to handle them.

Future Pacing

. . .

This is another technique that you can work with where you will ask a person to imagine that they are doing something in the future, and then you will monitor the reaction that they have to this. It is typically something that is going to be used in order to check that a change process has been successful. You can check this out by observing the body language of the target when this person is going through a difficult situation before and also after the intervention.

If you are doing this and notice that the body language is the same, then you know right away that the intervention has not been successful the way that you would like.

Future pacing is a technique that is going to help you to embed change into the contexts of what is going to happen in the future for that other individual. It gives a person the experience of dealing with a situation in a more positive manner before they have to go through and deal with that same situation in reality. This method is going to be based on the ideas and methods that come with visualization, where the mind is going to be assumed to not have the ability to tell the difference between when a situation is real, and one that has been visualized in a clear manner.

The theory of this is that, once the person has taken the

time to visualize the experience in a positive way, when they do actually encounter the situation, the visualized situation that they did before is going to be their model for how to behave in that situation, even those they only imagined and made up the visualization. The mind is not really able to come up with the differences between the real-life scenario and the imagined one, which can help the person to get through that whole situation much easier.

So, how is this going to be useful for the person who is trying to work with dark NLP? If you are worried about a specific situation, then the idea of future pacing is going to be able to help you out here. Before entering into that situation, take some time to visualize it in your head. Think about it in a positive way, imagining what it will feel like if that situation goes really well, above your own expectations, and if you were able to get through it without a hitch?

Try to imagine this as clearly as possible. Let's say that you are anxious about a job interview. Imagine what you are going to wear to the interview, what time you will show up, what you will say about your resume and the answers that you are going to give to the questions that you are asked. Imagine that you are shaking the hand of the person interviewing you and that you feel really good about the whole situation like you are sure that they will offer you the job because they were dazzled by your credentials and all of the things that you said during the interview.

You will find that if you were able to come up with a strong enough and clear enough picture and visualization of the event, that when you actually head to the real event, it won't seem so scary. Your brain will assume that it has already gone through all of this, and the situation is going to pan out much better than you would imagine.

Content reframing

The next thing that we need to take a look at is content reframing. This is another technique that you can use any time that you feel that the situation that is around you seems to be helpless or negative. When you take the time to reframe things, it is going to take away any of the negative out of the situation that you see, and it will empower you by changing the meaning of the experience into something that is going to feel and appear to be more positive to you.

A good example of this is to say that you were in a long relationship and then it ends. You may not have been the one to end it, and maybe the other person blindsided you with the news. When you take a look at this breakup on the surface, it is going to seem awful and all that you will want to do is go and sulk in all of the misery that you feel. But maybe the one thing that you need to focus on here is how to reframe the situation.

For example, what are some of the benefits that you could enjoy now that you are single? You could look at it as the ability to be open to a new, and hopefully better, relationship. You now have the ability to go and do what you want, when you want it, without having to worry about how it will affect the other person or what they are going to think about this newfound freedom. And after that relationship is over, you are able to take some of the valuable lessons that you learned from it along the way and use it to make sure that you have better and stronger relationships in the future.

There are a lot of ways that you are able to go through and reframe the situations around you. There are always going to be situations that are a bit negative, ones that don't seem to work the way that you want, and ones that will drag you down and make it seem hard to get the results that you want. But by simply looking at the positives of that situation, and there are always some things that are positive, and ignoring the negatives that can come with it, you can really start to see that the situation is not that bad.

. . .

In some situations, you will start to panic, or even focus on the fear that shows up. And this is pretty natural. But if you don't move the mind away from this panic and fear, it is just going to lead you to a lot more problems down the line, more things that you need to deal with. In contrast, when you shift your focus, using some of the ideas that we were talking about above, you will be able to clear out your head, and really think about whether the situation was as bad as you had first thought.

Anchoring yourself

The next method that we are going to explore is going to be that of anchoring. We spent a little bit of time talking about anchoring in this guidebook but didn't get a chance to go too much in depth about how it works, why you would use it and more. Now it is our chance to see some of the great things that you can do with the method of anchoring, and why it is one of the best methods to help you form a good connection with the other person.

The idea of anchoring is going to find its origins with Russian scientist Ivan Pavlov. Pavlov is well known for some of his experiments with dogs by ringing a bell repeatedly while those dogs were eating. After he repeated the ringing of the bell, Pavlov them found that simply by ringing the bell, even if he didn't bring out the food at that time, he was able to get the dogs to salivate. This was all just from hearing the bell.

The reason for this is that Pavlov had been able to create a big connection in the brain between the bell, and the behavior that would necessitate the salivating, namely, the eating of food. Then, when the dogs did hear the bell again, they assumed that food was on the way, or at least their brains did, and so the salivating started to prepare them for eating, even though there wasn't any food coming their way.

The neat thing about all of this is that you are able to use this same idea in order to stimulate a response that is anchored back to you. Instead of having the noise or the touch or other signal go back to food or something else, you are able to use it in a way that anchors your target right back to you.

Anchoring yourself is going to make sure that you associate the desired positive emotional response to a specific sensation or phrase that you choose. If you are able to choose the right kind of thought or emotion that is positive, and you are able to deliberately go through and connect it to a simple thought or gesture, you can then make sure that this anchor is triggered when you are feeling low. Then, you can do this gesture in order to help change around the feelings that you are dealing with.

1. The first thing to consider is what you would like to feel. You can pretty much anchor any kind of emotion that you would like, but most people are going to go with a good feeling like calmness, happiness, and confidence.
2. Decide where you want the anchor place to be on your body. You can pick almost anywhere but many times people like to squeeze on a fingernail, touch their knuckles, pull on the earlobe or even just touch their wrist. It is important to add some kind of physical touch to this because it allows you to trigger that positive feeling no matter when or where. The placement doesn't matter. But you want to make sure that it is unique enough that you aren't as likely to touch it randomly at any other point.
3. Think about a time in the past when you felt that state that you want to feel now. So, if you want to have more confidence, think back to a time in your

life when you felt you had a good deal of confidence.

4. Mentally go back to that time and float into your body. Look through your eyes of that moment, and relive the memory as much as you can. You can work to adjust your own body language so that it works with the memory. See what you saw, hear what you heard, and try to feel the feelings as much as you can and so on. This can help you to feel more in that state than ever before.

5. As you go back and relive some of that memory more and more, try to touch, pull, or squeeze the part of the body that you choose. You will feel that feeling swell as you go through and relive the memory. You can release the touch that the emotional state starts to reach its peak, and when it starts to wear off.

6. Doing this may seem a little silly when you first get started, but the point of doing this is to create a neurological stimulus response that is going to be able to trigger the emotion or the state at any time that you would like. If you have done this in the proper manner, you will be able to touch yourself and use the same pressure again in the future, and that emotion and that state will come back to you.

It is possible to do some steps in order to make the response even a little bit stronger. To do this, you can take the time to think about another memory, but make sure that this memory is about that same state that you wanted in the beginning. So if confidence was your goal to start, then think about a second memory where you felt confident.

Once you have that second memory, go back through it and relive it through your own eyes. Make sure that the anchor part of the body ends up being in the same spot that it was before. The more memories that you are able to add to this, and the stronger those memories are, the better off you will be. This anchor is going to become more potent, and even a single touch can be enough to trigger the response that you want. Aim to get in at least two or three memories to make this work, especially ones that are particularly strong. But if you are able to find more, you will be able to get an even stronger response in the process.

You can use this idea with dark NLP as well. You don't have to just use it on yourself. Many masters of NLP have been able to use this anchoring idea to work with other people and getting them anchored towards the manipulator. For example, if you want to make sure that someone sees you like something that makes them laugh or someone they feel comfortable with, you can use some of the steps above to create an anchor.

We talked about this a bit before, but say that you want to associate a good feeling that the target has back to you. You can start anchoring them each time that they laugh or feel good about themselves. Let's say that each time they laugh at one of your jokes, or at anything else that is going on, you touch them a bit, or even touch your wrist. Over time, you will be able to touch your wrist, even without the laughter, and induce some good feelings in the target without even needing to try in the process.

Getting other people to like you

One of the best things that you can do to make sure that others are going to be willing to do what you want, is to make sure that they like you. If you are likable, people are going to be more than willing to jump in and do what you want, without feeling like you are forcing them to do the action. It can take some time and some practice to get to this point, and you will have to take some special steps to make sure that you appear as likable as possible to that person. But once you are able to do it, you will be amazed at the results that you can get, and how willing they are to work with you.

Building up a rapport and making sure that other people, especially your target, like you, is one of the easier sets of NLP techniques that you can work with, but they can really make a difference. And these techniques are going to ensure that you are able to get along with pretty much anyone. The good news is that even if you are shy or have trouble talking to others, there are a lot of different methods that you can use in order to build up some of that rapport that you want with the other person.

One of the fastest, and often seen as one of the most effec- tive, methods to help you build up this rapport with the other person is to use the mirroring option. This is when you are going to subtly mirror the words, tone of voice, body language, and actions of the other person. This may seem simple, but it is really going to work to get the target to like you more and to be drawn to you more, even though they aren't even going to realize what is going on in the process.

People like to be around those who are like themselves. They find that when someone is too different from them, it can make them feel uncomfortable, and they may feel like they and the other person don't really have anything in common, or anything to talk about in the process. When you mirror the other person, making sure to be as subtle as possible with this, the brain is going to start firing off mirror neurons, which can be pleasure sensors that show up in the brain, and will make people sense a liking for the person who is mirroring them.

It is such a great way to make sure the other person likes you. Their subconscious is going to take note of the fact that you are talking like them, acting like them, and using the same body language as your target. This will make it so that the brain feels like there is a real connection going on there, and it is going to help the person to like you. In the process, since this is going on in the subconscious mind, the target isn't really going to realize what is going on. All they will know is that they find you to be really likable.

The technique of mirroring is going to be pretty simple. You will want to stand or sit the way that your target is sitting. If you see that they are tilting their head in one direction or another, you will want to make sure the head is tilted in the same manner. Smile when the target decides to smile, try to mirror the facial expressions, cross your legs if the other person seems to be doing that, try to mirror the voice and the tone they are using and more.

Of course, if you are using this method as a way to build up some of the rapport that you want, you must make sure that everything you are doing is done in a subtle manner. If you are too noticeable with the actions that you are taking, it is more likely that the other person is going to notice what is going on. And while you are doing it to make the target notice and like you, the target may think that you are mimicking them or making fun of them. This will break the rapport that you are trying to build up. Instead, make sure that any of the actions that you use with mirroring are kept minimal and that they stay as natural and calm in front of the other person as possible.

Using persuasion and influence

While we do spend a lot of time working with NLP in a way that is dedicated to helping people get rid of some of their negative emotions, limit their bad habits, beliefs, and conflict to name a few, another way that you can work with NLP is to spend some time figuring out how you can ethically persuade and influence other people.

. . .

One of the names in NLP that we haven't had time to talk about yet was someone known as Milton H. Erickson. He was a psychiatrist who spent some time studying how the subconscious mind worked and how it behaved when hypnotherapy happened. He spent this time working on how hypnotherapy could actually influence the brain, not the kind of stuff that we see in the movies or read about in books.

Erickson was actually so good at hypnosis that he was actually able to develop a new way to speak to the subconscious minds of other people, without even needing to place them in a state of hypnosis to start with. This means that he was able to go in and almost hypnotize a person at any time, and in any place, that he wanted, with just using what we would consider regular and everyday kinds of conversation in the process. This actually developed into its own form of hypnosis and is known as conversational hypnosis today.

This is actually a powerful tool that someone can use in order to not only persuade and influence the others who are around them all the time, but to make sure that the target is able to overcome some of the fears that they have, some of their limiting beliefs, conflict and more without their conscious awareness. This is going to be more useful when getting across to people who might otherwise be resistant if they knew what is going on with what you are saying.

As you can see, there are a lot of different techniques that you can use when it comes to implementing NLP in your life. Each of these is going to work in a slightly different manner to ensure that you are able to reach the target, or even improve yourself, and see some amazing results. Start practicing with a few of these methods and options in order to see which one you like the best, and then choose the one that works based on the situation you find yourself in.

Conclusion

Thank for making it through to the end of NLP, let's hope it was informative and able to provide you with all of the tools you need to achieve your goals whatever they may be.

The next step is to start implementing some of the techniques and ideas that we have discussed in this guidebook into your own life. Anyone is able to learn how to work with NLP. It is not a secret that is just meant for some. The problem is that too many people are held back by not understanding what NLP is all about and they may decide that their morals don't allow for this kind of behavior. Because of this, they are going to shy away from even hearing about NLP, despite all of the benefits that this can bring to them.

This puts you at a distinct advantage over the others. You will be able to utilize the skills that we discussed in this guidebook to your own advantage, using the skills and some of the other options that we talked about, in order to make sure that you get what you want from those who are in your life. And since most people aren't expecting this to occur to them, you are going to end up being the winner in the long run.

When you are ready to learn a little bit more about NLP, especially when it comes to dark NLP< make sure to use this guidebook to make sure that you get started on the right track.

Finally, if you found this book useful in any way, a review on Amazon is always appreciated!

Milton Keynes UK
Ingram Content Group UK Ltd.
UKHW020648070923
428221UK00013B/71

9 781087 863887